Patient Billing

... Using **MEDISOFT FOR WINDOWS**

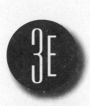

Greg Harpole

Oregon State Department of Education

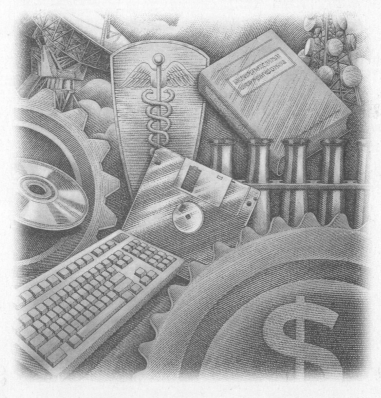

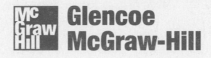 **Glencoe McGraw-Hill**

New York, New York   Columbus, Ohio   Woodland Hills, California   Peoria, Illinois

Patient Billing: Using MediSoft for Windows, **Third Edition**

ISBN: 0-02-8012410

Library of Congress Cataloging-in-Publication Data

Harpole, Greg.
    Patient billing : using MediSoft for Windows / Greg Harpole. --
3rd ed.
        p.   cm.
    Includes windows.
    ISBN 0-02-801241-0 (text with disk). -- ISBN 0-02-801242-9
(instructor's manual with disk)
    1. MediSoft. 2. Medical fees--Computer programs.   3. Collecting
of accounts--Computer programs.   I. Title.
R728.5.H378   1997   97-51749
610'.681--dc21   CIP

Microsoft and *Windows* are registered trademarks of *Microsoft Corporation.*
MediSoft is a registered trademark of *MediSoft, Inc.*

Send all inquiries to:
Glencoe/McGraw-Hill
8787 Orion Place
Columbus, OH 43240

4 5 6 7 8 9 10 11 12 13 14 15   009   04 03 02 01 00

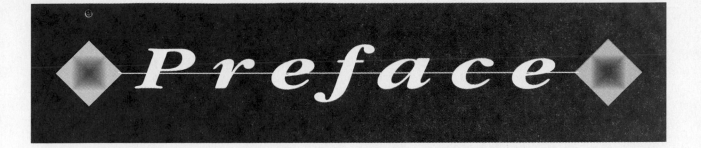

Health care continues to be one of the fastest growing industries. As such, there is increasing need for both health care professionals and support staff. One important support function involves the accounting and patient billing aspects of a medical practice. Although the accounting requirements have become steadily more complex, individuals who have practical experience using patient billing software are more suited for these challenging tasks. Anyone who aims to get a job as a medical billing assistant will find that an understanding of computer technology is often a prerequisite to being hired.

This text/workbook, *Patient Billing: A Computerized Simulation Using MediSoft for Windows*, will help prepare you to perform the duties of a medical billing assistant. It combines a step-by-step tutorial with a comprehensive simulation. In the tutorial, you will learn how to use *MediSoft* (a widely used patient accounting program) to perform the following tasks:

◆ Add new billing codes

◆ Input patient information

◆ Process patient transactions

◆ Produce various reports

◆ Print statements and insurance forms

◆ Process claims

The tutorial also provides an overview of the medical office accounting procedures, introduces you to the features of a patient billing system, and presents important concepts relating to a medical office accounting function.

After you learn the basic patient billing tasks, the simulation lets you practice the skills you have learned. In the simulation, you will assume the role of a medical billing assistant in a doctor's office. You will use the *MediSoft* program to process a variety of billing transactions for an entire week. By the time you complete the simulation, you will have mastered many of the medical billing skills that are highly regarded and sought after in the health care profession.

While this text/workbook features the *MediSoft* program, the concepts introduced are general enough to cover most patient billing and accounting software. After you complete the tutorial and simulation provided in this text/workbook, you should be able to use almost any such software available, even custom software, with a minimum of training.

COMPONENTS

Patient Billing: A Computerized Simulation Using MediSoft for Windows consists of a text/workbook and a student data disk. The text/workbook thoroughly explains new concepts and provides step-by-step instructions that help you learn how to use the *MediSoft* program. The student data disk contains all of the data needed to perform patient billing activities for the Family Care Center—a small medical practice. You will not waste time entering basic information such as existing patients, diagnosis codes, and procedure codes. With the student data disk, you can immediately focus on learning how to use the *MediSoft* program.

FEATURES

Patient Billing: A Computerized Simulation Using MediSoft for Windows includes many special features designed to help you master the *MediSoft* billing software. The major features are the following:

◆ The text/workbook is divided into two separate sections— tutorial and simulation. The tutorial lets you learn the basic *MediSoft* software features and the simulation helps you master the program.

◆ The tutorial thoroughly describes all of the *MediSoft* options and features that relate to patient billing. To help you understand these new concepts, the tutorial uses the Family Care Center as a realistic medical office setting in which you perform many of the tasks.

◆ Step-by-step instructions guide you through each new activity. Practice exercises begin with simple tasks and progress to more complex activities throughout the tutorial.

◆ The tutorial includes many screen illustrations, source documents, and sample reports to reinforce the concepts introduced in the text/workbook.

◆ Reminders or tips are placed throughout the tutorial. These tips identify shortcuts and list other helpful information for using the *MediSoft* program more effectively.

◆ After you finish the tutorial, a comprehensive simulation lets you step into the role of billing assistant for the Family Care Center. You will assume the responsibility for all medical billing activities during a week in September. As you complete the simulation, you will add new patients, create cases, process procedure charges, enter payments, print reports, and handle claims.

RESOURCES FOR THE INSTRUCTOR

Teaching students how to use a software application such as *MediSoft* can be a challenging endeavor. If you have never taught this course or if you are upgrading from the MS-DOS version to the *Windows* version, your job is even more challenging. That's why the instructor's manual includes tips, suggestions, and comprehensive information for getting started with the *MediSoft* program.

After you install the software and are ready for your students to begin using the *MediSoft* program, you can rely on the manual for important information that you can use to help your students work through the tutorial. The manual includes chapter-by-chapter teaching suggestions, checkpoint answers, end-of-chapter solutions, and sample printouts corresponding to the practice exercises. Numerous printouts and solutions for the simulation are also provided so that you can check your students' work every step of the way or after they have finished the simulation.

A student data disk is packaged with the manual for your convenience. You can use the disk to explore the *MediSoft* application software yourself, or you can make the data disk available to your students in the event they need to start over.

The manual also includes other information and resources that will help you effectively teach your students how to use the *MediSoft* program. These resources include transparency masters for many of the *MediSoft* screens and troubleshooting tips that may prove helpful if you experience problems using the billing software.

ACKNOWLEDGMENTS ➤

Sincere appreciation is expressed to the following reviewers for their thoughtful suggestions and careful checking of this edition: Jeff Ward (*MediSoft*, Mesa, Arizona); Wanda Card (Pitt Community College, Greenville, North Carolina); and Tabitha Ratcliffe (Columbus State Community College, Columbus, Ohio).

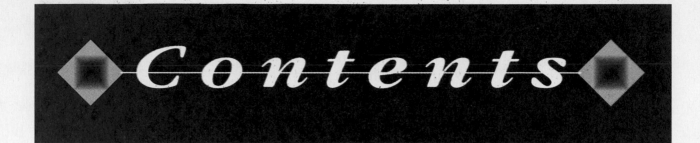

FAMILY CARE CENTER—A PATIENT BILLING SIMULATION 147

INTRODUCTION

OVERVIEW

MediSoft is a popular patient billing and accounting software program. It enables health care practices to maintain their billing data as well as to generate report information. The software handles all the basic tasks that a medical billing assistant needs to effectively perform his/her job. As such, *MediSoft* is an excellent training tool for anyone interested in working as a medical billing assistant. Even if you do not use *MediSoft* on the job, the skills you learn here will be similar to those skills needed to use almost any medical accounting program.

This text/workbook includes a tutorial and a comprehensive simulation. Once you learn how to operate the *MediSoft* program by completing the tutorial, you can practice those skills by working through the simulation. Both the tutorial and the simulation use a medical office setting, Family Care Center, to provide a realistic environment in which you can learn how to use the software.

GETTING STARTED

Before you jump into the tutorial, review the information provided in this Getting Started section. Here you will find information that describes the setting and explains your role as a medical billing assistant at the Family Care Center. This section also includes a description of how this text/workbook is organized, start-up instructions for the *MediSoft* program, and tips for using the accompanying student data disk.

Family Care Center

Dr. Katherine Yan, for whom you will work, operates the Family Care Center located in the Stephenson Medical Complex. This medical complex includes suites for 27 doctors, a pharmacy, and a laboratory with X-ray equipment. Like the other medical practices at the Stephenson Medical Complex, the Family Care Center is independently run. Referrals, however, are often made among the physicians in the complex.

Dr. Yan's Office   Dr. Katherine Yan specializes in family practice, which means she is qualified to treat infants, children, and adults. She treats a wide variety of medical conditions such as gynecological problems, cardiac problems, infections, and fractures. Dr. Yan is the first doctor her patients consult for almost any medical problem and for routine physical checkups as well. When patients need more specialized care, such as surgery or obstetrical services for the birth of a baby, Dr. Yan refers her patients to other doctors. Since a variety of specialists have offices in the complex, Dr. Yan is able to send most of her patients to other physicians there. In return, she sees patients who are referred to her by other doctors in the complex.

The office suite that Dr. Yan leases is located just off the landscaped courtyard in the center of the medical complex. Parking is nearby, providing easy access to the office for the physically handicapped patients. The office suite (Figure I-1, page 3) consists of the following rooms:

♦ A reception area with comfortable furniture and reading materials for adults and children. The office receptionist sits at a workstation in this area. Patients check in here when they arrive and make appointments and pay bills here when they leave. This is where the main office phone is located. The appointment book is kept near the phone so that the receptionist can schedule appointments when patients call the office.

♦ A spacious office off the reception area with a desk for the medical billing assistant, a computer, a variety of office equipment, and a wall of file drawers. Patient charts, patient financial and medical records, and other records are stored in this area. There is a phone in this area as well, so that the medical billing assistant can handle inquiries from patients and phone calls to patients and insurance companies about their bills and unpaid claims.

♦ An office for the office manager, next to the medical billing assistant's office.

♦ An adjacent hallway leading to the following rooms within the office suite: minor surgery room, three examination rooms, small laboratory for routine tests (other tests are performed at the laboratory in the medical complex), office where Dr. Yan speaks with patients, supply room with medical and office supplies, and a rest room.

The office is open Monday, Tuesday, Wednesday, and Friday from 8:30 a.m. to noon and 1:30 to 5:00 p.m. On Thursday the office hours

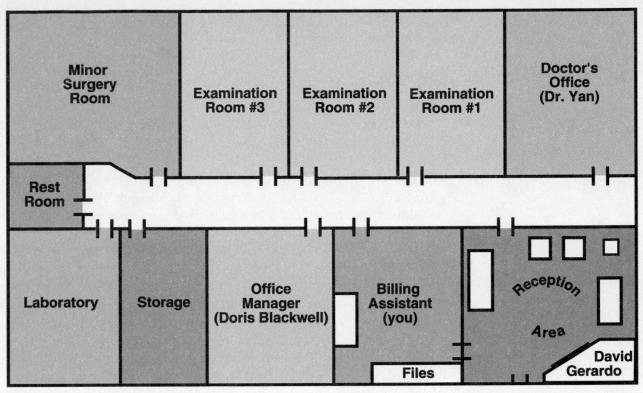

Figure I-1 *Family Care Center Floor Plan*

are 8:30 a.m. to noon. Dr. Yan shares nonoffice-hour calls with six other doctors in the area. She is on call Tuesday evenings and every seventh weekend for emergencies. When Dr. Yan is on call, the members of her staff are also asked to be available in case they are needed.

Members of Dr. Yan's staff include:

◆ Doris Blackwell—Office Manager. Doris has been with the doctor for the past four years and supervises the business aspects of the practice. She also serves as the accountant for the office, doing payroll, accounts payable, and so on, working closely with a certified public accountant.

◆ Michelle Walcott—Clinical Assistant. Michelle has worked with Dr. Yan for the past six years. She prepares patients to see the doctor, gives injections, changes dressings, assists in minor surgery, and generally helps the doctor with patient care.

◆ David Gerardo—Receptionist/Administrative Medical Office Assistant. David handles the front desk and the phones, pulls patients' charts for daily appointments, files the charts, schedules appointments, and orders supplies.

◆ You—Medical Billing Assistant. Dr. Yan has recently hired you as the new medical billing assistant to replace Bill Larson, who has moved out of the area. Your first responsibility is to learn the *MediSoft* patient billing and accounting software. Although your primary responsibility is for patient records and patient billing, Dr. Yan wants to be sure that you are familiar with the basic accounting system used in the office. The office uses the cash basis for accounting, which means that all revenues are recorded when they are actually received and that expenses are recorded only when they are paid.

The patient billing portion of the accounting system has been computerized using *MediSoft Patient Accounting for Windows*. The remaining accounting tasks are performed manually using a journal and ledger system.

Your Role   Since one of your major responsibilities is to handle patient records in *MediSoft*, Dr. Yan has asked that you become familiar with *MediSoft* as soon as possible. You will begin your training by reading materials about how a medical office operates and about how a computerized patient billing system works. The materials will enable you to learn and practice using the various functions of the software before you work with real information.

After you have completed Chapters 1 through 7 of the instructional materials, you will enter patient information for Dr. Yan's office for a four-day period. This will give you an opportunity to work with actual patient information and to try out what you have learned.

How This Book Is Organized

Review the information presented here for an overview of how this text/workbook is organized. A brief description of the tutorial chapters and the simulation is provided.

Chapter 1 describes the functions of a patient billing system and explains how it fits into the overall accounting operation of a medical office.

Chapter 2 explains how a computerized billing system handles data and compares the computerized system to a manual system.

Chapter 3 introduces the basic procedures needed to handle data with a computerized system. It covers keyboarding skills, navigating through the menus, searching for information, and backing up and restoring data.

Chapters 4 through 7 cover the actual use of *MediSoft*, explaining and illustrating most of the major operations possible with the system.

The Patient Billing Simulation and the Procedures Manual follow the last chapter. The simulation contains the Family Care Center data for the period from September 8, 1998 to September 11, 1998.

The Procedures Manual provides instructions and helpful tips for using the *MediSoft* program.

When you work through a chapter, follow these steps:

♦ Read the text. Study the figures and screen illustrations that accompany the explanations of various topics.

♦ As you read, answer the Checkpoint questions that appear throughout the chapter. Write your answers in the text/work-book. Look back at the text if necessary to determine your answer.

♦ Throughout the tutorial, there are practice exercises that you must complete at the computer. Work through each practice exercise by following the step-by-step instructions. The source documents referred to in the practice exercises are located at the back of the book beginning on page 159.

♦ Do not skip any practice exercises. You must complete all of the exercises before you begin the simulation.

♦ If you experience difficulty completing a practice exercise, review the corresponding section in the tutorial and then try the exercise again.

♦ Complete the chapter review questions after you finish each chapter.

When you have finished Chapters 1 to 7, complete the Patient Billing Simulation by following the instructions beginning on page 147 of the text/workbook.

Making a Backup of Your Student Data Disk

Before you begin using the student data disk with the *MediSoft* soft-ware, make a backup copy of the disk. Label one disk "Working Copy" and the other disk "Original." If you accidentally damage your data disk or need to restart the simulation, you can make another copy of the original disk.

As you work through this tutorial and simulation, you should make a copy of your working disk at the end of each session. Use another disk—not the original disk—to make your backup copy.

Follow the instructions provided below to make a copy of the student data disk.

Windows 3.1

1. Insert the student data disk into a floppy disk drive.

2. Double-click the **File Manager** program icon.

3. Pull down the **Disk** menu and choose the *Copy Disk* option.

4. Set the source and the destination information. (The *source* is the disk drive to copy from; the *destination* is the disk drive to copy to.)

5. Click the **OK** button.

6. Store the original disk in a safe place.

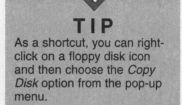

TIP

As a shortcut, you can right-click on a floppy disk icon and then choose the *Copy Disk* option from the pop-up menu.

Windows 95

1. Insert the student data disk into a floppy disk drive.

2. Double-click the **My Computer** icon shown on the Desktop.

3. Click the icon for the disk drive containing the disk that you want to copy.

4. Pull down the **File** menu and choose the *Copy Disk* option.

5. Choose the disk drive to copy from and the disk drive to copy to.

6. Click the **Start** button.

7. Store the original disk in a safe place.

Starting *MediSoft*

Follow the instructions provided here to start the *MediSoft for Windows* software.

1. Turn on the computer and insert your data disk into Drive A or B, whichever is appropriate.

> **IMPORTANT:** Never remove your data disk from the drive while the *MediSoft* program is running. Be sure to quit the program before you remove the data disk.

2. Refer to the appropriate instructions that correspond to your computer system. The program requires a few moments to start and open the practice data from the floppy disk drive.

   Windows 3.1: Locate the *MediSoft* program icon. Double-click the program icon to start the software.

   Windows 95: Click the **Start** button on the Taskbar. Highlight the **Programs** menu and locate the *MediSoft 5.2* folder. Select the *MediSoft* option to start the software.

3. Verify that the program opened the Family Care Center Practice data. The program name and current practice information (i.e., MediSoft—Family Care Center) appear at the top of the window. (See Figure I-2, page 7.)

Practice Name

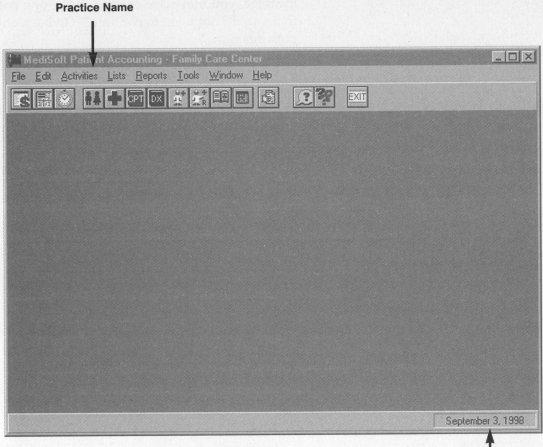

September 3, 1998

Figure I-2 *Family Care Center Opening Screen*

Current Date

If the program does not automatically open the Family Care Center, try to manually open or select the practice. Pull down the **File** menu and choose the *Open Practice* option. Select *Family Care Center* if it appears in the list. The program should read the information from your data disk.

If this is the first time you are using the *MediSoft* program or the practice information was removed, you may have to create a new practice before you can continue. Follow these steps to create a new practice.

◆ Click the **Create a new set of data** button if prompted, or choose the *New Practice* option from the File menu.

◆ Enter **Family Care Center** for the practice name and **A:\FAMILY** for the data path. (Use **B:\FAMILY** if your data disk is located in Drive B.)

◆ Click the **Create** button.

◆ When prompted that data already exists in this directory, click the **Yes** button to continue. If you don't see this message, you may have entered the wrong path. Indicate that you do not want to continue. Go back and enter the path again.

♦ Review the information in the Practice Information dialog box, then click the **Save** button to continue.

♦ Pull down the File menu and choose the Set Program Date option. Enter **September 3, 1998** for the date unless instructed otherwise in the tutorial or simulation. Be sure to enter the date correctly since *MediSoft* relies on the date to process information. You are now ready to begin using the software.

Chapter 1

INTRODUCTION TO PATIENT BILLING

WHAT YOU WILL LEARN

When you finish this chapter, you will be able to:

1. Define the terms introduced in this chapter.

2. Describe the major elements of a manual patient billing system.

3. Explain how patient billing fits into the overall accounting system.

4. Define the financial records a medical billing assistant maintains.

5. Discuss the day-to-day responsibilities of a medical billing assistant.

KEY TERMS

Case	A grouping of procedures or transactions generally organized by the type of treatment or insurance carrier.
Cash payments journal	Record of all cash payments, frequently in the form of a checkbook register.
Cash receipts journal	Record of all cash received by a business.
Champus and *CHAMP/VA*	Governmental health insurance plans for eligible dependents of military personnel and disabled veterans, respectively.
CPT-4	Listing of codes for medical services or procedures.
Day sheet	Daily record of activities, patients treated, fees charged, and payments received.
General ledger	Record of all the accounts of a business.
Guarantor	The person or third party responsible for payment of a patient's medical bills.

HCFA-1500	An insurance form accepted by governmental insurance plans in some states and by most private insurers. This form is required by Medicare nationwide.
ICD-9	Listing of codes for medical diagnoses.
Journal	Record of daily transactions listed in chronological order, also known as the book of original entry.
Ledger	A group of accounts where debits and credits are posted from the book of original entry.
Medicaid	Health insurance offered by the government for low-income people (in California, called Medi-Cal).
Medicare	Governmental health insurance made available to elderly and disabled people.
Patient ledger	Record of all activity (charges, payments, and adjustments) in an individual patient's account.
Procedure	A service performed by a physician or other provider.
Provider	The medical staff member, such as a doctor or physical therapist, who performs the various services.
Superbill	Record of one patient's visit, showing procedures performed, charges, and diagnosis. In a manual system, this document may also be referred to as a fee slip, routing slip, or encounter form.

OVERVIEW OF MEDICAL OFFICE ACCOUNTING

Like other businesses, a medical office must track the flow of money into and out of the practice. Keeping accurate financial records helps **providers**, the medical personnel who perform the various procedures, make sure that they are properly compensated for the services they perform. Financial data is also important for tax-reporting purposes and is useful in determining whether or not a practice is profitable.

Medical offices record their financial records in a series of journals and ledgers. A **journal** is a record of the daily transactions listed in chronological order, and a **ledger** shows the activity for each account. The **cash payments journal** lists payments made by check to vendors and employees; and the **cash receipts journal** is used to record any money received.

Patient billing, which involves tracking how much money patients owe and what they have paid, is a key part of a medical office accounting system. The patient billing duties are the primary responsibility of the medical billing assistant. To perform these duties, the billing assistant uses day sheets and patient ledgers. The **day sheet** (or general journal or daily journal) is a chronological record of all transactions involving patients. From the day sheet, information on the activity in each patient's account can be transferred to the appropriate **patient ledger**.

Once the billing assistant generates the patient ledgers, the accountant can use this information to update the general ledger. The **general ledger** includes up-to-date balances for all of a medical practice's accounts, and is used to prepare various financial statements, such as an income statement or balance sheet.

PATIENT BILLING

As a medical billing assistant, you will be responsible for all aspects of the patient billing process. On a daily basis, you will most likely maintain various records, enter payments, update patient ledgers, prepare patient statements, and process insurance claims along with other tasks.

This section describes how a billing assistant would perform his or her duties in a manual system without the aid of a computer. The next chapter discusses how a computerized accounting system can be used to make this process more efficient.

Records Kept by the Medical Billing Assistant

A billing assistant must maintain various records that are needed by a practice for it to operate smoothly. Review the information provided here that describes some of these records such as the superbill, patient cases, day sheets, and the patient ledger.

Superbill A **superbill** (or charge slip) is a paper document that lists all services performed for one patient at a single office visit. The form has places for the patient's name, medical services provided that day, diagnosis, amount of each individual charge for that day, total for the visit, and the amount paid. A **diagnosis** is the doctor's determination of what is wrong with the patient, based on an examination.

A sample superbill is shown in Figure 1-1, page 12. A superbill is attached to each patient's chart at the start of the visit. The doctor, lab technician, nurse, and anyone else who performs a procedure for the patient during that visit records the service on the superbill. A **procedure** is a service performed, such as an office visit with a doctor (including examination, evaluation of symptoms, and determination of a course of treatment), an injection, or a laboratory test. At the end of the visit, the assistant at the front desk uses the superbill to calculate the total charge and to record any payment received. The superbill then goes to the medical billing assistant, who uses it as the source document to update the patient ledger and the day sheet.

Family Care Center
285 Stephenson Boulevard
Stephenson, OH 60089
(614) 555-0100

Provider: Dr. Katherine Yan   **ID #:** 84021   **S.S. #:** 810-99-1110

Patient:	Chart #:	Document:
Address:	Phone:	Date:

CODE	DESCRIPTION	X
New Patient		
99201	OF—New Patient Focused	
99202	OF—New Patient Expanded	
99203	OF—New Patient, Complete Physical	
Established Patient		
99213	OF—Established Patient Expanded	
99214	OF—Established Patient Routine Exam	
99215	OF—Established Patient Complex	
99211	OF—Established Patient Minimal	
99212	OF—Established Patient Focused	
Procedures		
85007	Manual WBC	
85651	Erythrocyte Sed Rate—ESR	
86403	Strep Test, Rapid	
86585	Tine Test	
87072	Strep Culture	
87086	Urine Culture	
93000	Electroencephalogram—EEG	
93015	Treadmill Stress Test	
90782	Injection	
Other Procedures		

Payments:
Diagnosis/ICD-9:

Remarks:	Today's Charges: $
Next Appointment:	Amount Paid: $

Figure 1-1 *Sample Superbill*

Case Many medical offices organize patient records using a case-based system. That is, all patient payments, insurance claim reimbursements, and adjustments are linked to a case. A **case** is a grouping of procedures or transactions generally organized by the type of treatment or insurance carrier. For every new case, a billing assistant must record the pertinent information including the following: case description, guarantor, marital status, employer, provider, insurance carrier, policy number, and diagnosis. The **guarantor** is the person or party responsible for payment of a patient's medical bills.

Day Sheet The **day sheet** is a list of patients, charges, and services performed each day. In a manual system, a billing assistant must prepare the day sheet from the individual superbills and case reports. Day sheets have columns with headings such as "Entry," "Date," "Document," "Description," "Provider," "Code," and "Amount." New charges, payments, adjustments, and the current balance are shown for each patient. A summary of the day's activity appears at the end of the report. (See the sample day sheet in Figure 1-2, page 14.)

Patient Ledger The **patient ledger** is used to track, or show, all the activity for each patient account. To complete this ledger, a billing assistant must manually gather the required information from the superbills and day sheet. Since some patients do not pay when services are provided, it is very important that the office keep a record of how much each patient owes. The patient ledger report serves two purposes:

◆ an internal record that shows the amount each patient owes; and

◆ patient statement of account, or bill.

A sample patient ledger is illustrated in Figure 1-3, page 15. The patient ledger report includes the patient's name, procedure date and code, provider, charges, payments, adjustments, and the account balance.

C H E C K P O I N T

1. Which form is also referred to as a charge slip?

   Superbill

2. Which ledger is used to track all of the activity for a patient?

   Patient Ledger

3. Which report shows the patients seen, charges recorded, and services performed each day?

   Day Sheet

Family Care Center
Patient Day Sheet

Entry	Date	Document	POS	Description	Provider	Code	Amount
BAREL000	**Ellen Barmenstein**						
1	8/28/98	9808280000	11		1	99212	60.00
2	8/28/98	9808280000				01	-20.00
		Today's Charges		Today's Receipts	Adjustments		Patient Balance
		$60.00		-$20.00	$0.00		$40.00
BELHE000	**Herbert Bell**						
3	8/28/98	9808280000	11		1	99212	60.00
4	8/28/98	9808280000	11		1	93015	150.00
5	8/28/98	9808280000				02	-60.00
		Today's Charges		Today's Receipts	Adjustments		Patient Balance
		$210.00		-$60.00	$0.00		$150.00
JONEL000	**Elizabeth Jones**						
16	8/28/98	9808280000	11		1	99212	60.00
17	8/28/98	9808280000	11		1	90782	10.00
		Today's Charges		Today's Receipts	Adjustments		Patient Balance
		$70.00		$0.00	$0.00		$70.00

Total Procedure Charges	$340.00
Total Product Charges	$0.00
Total Inside Lab Charges	$0.00
Total Outside Lab Charges	$0.00
Total Insurance Payments	$0.00
Total Cash Co-payments	$0.00
Total Check Co-payments	$0.00
Total Credit Card Co-payments	$0.00
Total Patient Cash Payments	-$20.00
Total Patient Check Payments	-$60.00
Total Credit Card Payments	$0.00
Total Deductibles	$0.00
Total Credit Adjustments	$0.00
Total Debit Adjustments	$0.00
Total Medicare Debit Adjustments	$0.00
Total Medicare Credit Adjustments	$0.00
Net Effect on Accounts Receivable	$260.00

Figure 1-2 *Sample Day Sheet*

| | | | Family Care Center | | | | |
| | | | Patient Account Ledger | | | | |

Entry	Date	POS	Description	Procedure	Document	Provider	Amount
BAREL000	Ellen Barmenstein		(614)274-4242				
	Last Payment: -20.00		On: 8/28/98				
1	8/28/98	11		99212	9808280000	1	60.00
2	8/28/98			01	9808280000		-20.00
		Patient Totals					$40.00
BELHE000	Herbert Bell		(614)241-6124				
	Last Payment: -60.00		On: 8/28/98				
3	8/28/98	11		99212	9808280000	1	60.00
4	8/28/98	11		93015	9808280000	1	150.00
5	8/28/98			02	9808280000		-60.00
		Patient Totals					$150.00
BRORA000	Rachel Brown		(614)721-0044				
	Last Payment:		On:				
9	8/22/98	11		99211	9808280000	1	50.00
10	8/22/98	11		83718	9808280000	1	25.00
		Patient Totals					$75.00
JONEL000	Elizabeth Jones		(614)321-5555				
	Last Payment:		On:				
16	8/28/98	11		99212	9808280000	1	60.00
17	8/28/98	11		90782	9808280000	1	10.00
		Patient Totals					$70.00
MITHE000	Herbert Mitchell		(614)861-0909				
	Last Payment:		On:				
20	8/25/98	11		99213	9808280000	1	105.00
		Patient Totals					$105.00
WONLI000	Li Yu Wong		(614)751-7677				
	Last Payment:		On:				
46	8/20/98	11		99212	9808280000	1	60.00
47	8/20/98	11		90782	9808280000	1	5.00
		Patient Totals					$65.00
		Ledger Total					$505.00

Figure 1-3 *Sample Patient Ledger*

Day-to-Day Activities

As a billing assistant, your job is to follow a routine each day to keep the patient accounts up to date. Throughout the month, you must also send out patient statements and process insurance claims.

Recording Information   On a daily basis, a billing assistant uses the superbills to record case information, identify procedure charges, process patient payments, and make account adjustments. To simplify the billing process, medical offices use a set of standard procedure codes known as **CPT-4** (Current Procedural Terminology). Procedures that are commonly performed in the practice are usually listed on the superbill along with the corresponding CPT-4 code. For example, the sample superbill shown in Figure 1-1 includes several procedure codes such as 86403 (rapid strep test) and 90782 (injection). A doctor would mark these two codes if he or she administered a quick strep test and then gave the patient an injection of an antibiotic.

As part of the patient case information, you must also record the diagnosis. A set of medical diagnosis codes known as **ICD-9** (International Classification of Diseases, 9th edition) makes this task much easier. For instance, if a doctor wrote "strep throat" on a patient's superbill, you would use the code for strep throat (034.0) to record this diagnosis.

Entering Payments   Every day, as a billing assistant, you will record all payments received from patients and their insurance carriers. You will record these receipts on a day sheet and the appropriate patient ledgers.

Preparing the Bank Deposit   In some medical offices, you may also have the responsibility to prepare a bank deposit slip. Each day you will record all of the checks and cash received on a deposit slip, and then take the deposit to the bank. To verify that you recorded the day's receipts correctly, you can compare the bank deposit total with the day sheet total. Both totals should match.

Preparing Patient Statements   Usually, a billing assistant prepares and mails patient statements once a month. The statements summarize the office visits and charges during the month, itemize payments on the account, and show the unpaid account balance. The statement is the patient's bill for services. In some practices, statements are sent on several days during each month. For example, patients whose last names begin with *A* to *M* may be billed on the 15th of the month and patients with last names beginning with *N* to *Z* may be billed on the last day of the month. Spreading out the billing means there is less work to be done on one day, and payments from patients will be distributed more evenly throughout the month.

Preparing Insurance Forms Very few patients pay all of their medical bills themselves. Most people have some kind of medical insurance to help cover the costs. Some patients file their own insurance claims, often attaching a copy of the superbill to their claim form. Increasingly, however, medical offices file insurance claim forms directly with carriers. It is the medical billing assistant's job to be sure that those forms are filled out correctly and sent to insurance carriers and to record payments that come in directly to the office from the carriers. In addition to indicating the CPT-4 code and charges on the insurance form, you will enter some basic information about the patient, and a code for the diagnosis.

Types of Insurance Carriers The following table shows the principal types of insurance carriers that you will deal with.

CARRIER	DESCRIPTION
Blue Cross/Blue Shield	Nonprofit plans with medical, surgical, and hospital benefits. Payments are often made directly to the provider.
Commercial Insurers	Profit-making medical, surgical, and hospitalization insurance plans. Payments are often made directly to the patient.
Medicare	Governmental health insurance for the elderly. Part A covers hospital services. Part B partially pays for doctor's services. Payments are made to the provider in most cases.
Medicaid (Medi–Cal)	Governmental health insurance for low-income people. Payments are made to the provider.
Champus and CHAMP/VA	Governmental health insurance for dependents of certain military personnel (Champus) and dependents of disabled veterans (CHAMP/VA). Payments are made to the provider.
Health Maintenance Organization (HMO)	A medical center or group of providers that provides medical services to the patient for a fixed yearly fee. Providers are paid salaries.
Preferred Provider Organization (PPO)	Insurer contracts with a group of providers who agree to provide care based on a predetermined list of charges. The provider bills the PPO directly.

Table 1-1 *Types of Insurance Carriers*

Most governmental insurance plans and most private carriers accept a standard insurance form, the HCFA-1500. (See Figure 1-4, page 19.) Some private carriers require that their own claim form be used.

In addition, you may deal with workers' compensation, a state-regulated type of insurance covering certain on-the-job injuries.

Maintaining Patient Information

When a new patient comes to the office for the first time, he or she fills out a patient information form that asks for the following information: patient's name, address, employer, insurance coverage, marital status, and so on. When a patient moves, changes jobs, changes insurance carriers, or has other new information, that information must be entered on a patient information form as well. As the medical billing assistant, you must make sure that new and updated information is used in preparing insurance forms and statements.

C H E C K P O I N T

4. What reference is used to find a procedure code?

CPT-4

5. What reference can be used to find a list of common diagnoses?

ICD9

6. What type of form is typically used to process insurance claims?

HCFA - 1500

PLEASE
DO NOT
STAPLE
IN THIS
AREA

CARRIER →

HEALTH INSURANCE CLAIM FORM

PICA   PICA

1. MEDICARE	MEDICAID	CHAMPUS	CHAMPVA	GROUP HEALTH PLAN	FECA BLK LUNG	OTHER	1a. INSURED'S I.D. NUMBER (FOR PROGRAM IN ITEM 1)
(Medicare#)	(Medicaid #)	(Sponsor's SSN)	(VA File #)	(SSN or ID)	(SSN)	(ID)	

2. PATIENT'S NAME (Last Name, First Name, Middle Initial)

3. PATIENT'S BIRTH DATE   MM   DD   YY   SEX   M   F

4. INSURED'S NAME (Last Name, First Name, Middle Initial)

5. PATIENT'S ADDRESS (No., Street)

6. PATIENT RELATIONSHIP TO INSURED   Self   Spouse   Child   Other

7. INSURED'S ADDRESS (No., Street)

CITY   STATE

8. PATIENT STATUS   Single   Married   Other

CITY   STATE

ZIP CODE   TELEPHONE (Include Area Code)   (   )

Employed   Full-Time Student   Part-Time Student

ZIP CODE   TELEPHONE (INCLUDE AREA CODE)   (   )

9. OTHER INSURED'S NAME (Last Name, First Name, Middle Initial)

10. IS PATIENT'S CONDITION RELATED TO:

11. INSURED'S POLICY GROUP OR FECA NUMBER

a. OTHER INSURED'S POLICY OR GROUP NUMBER

a. EMPLOYMENT? (CURRENT OR PREVIOUS)   YES   NO

a. INSURED'S DATE OF BIRTH   MM   DD   YY   SEX   M   F

b. OTHER INSURED'S DATE OF BIRTH   MM   DD   YY   SEX   M   F

b. AUTO ACCIDENT?   PLACE (State)   YES   NO

b. EMPLOYER'S NAME OR SCHOOL NAME

c. EMPLOYER'S NAME OR SCHOOL NAME

c. OTHER ACCIDENT?   YES   NO

c. INSURANCE PLAN NAME OR PROGRAM NAME

d. INSURANCE PLAN NAME OR PROGRAM NAME

10d. RESERVED FOR LOCAL USE

d. IS THERE ANOTHER HEALTH BENEFIT PLAN?   YES   NO   *If yes,* return to and complete item 9 a-d.

READ BACK OF FORM BEFORE COMPLETING & SIGNING THIS FORM.
12. PATIENT'S OR AUTHORIZED PERSON'S SIGNATURE I authorize the release of any medical or other information necessary to process this claim. I also request payment of government benefits either to myself or to the party who accepts assignment below.

SIGNED _____   DATE _____

13. INSURED'S OR AUTHORIZED PERSON'S SIGNATURE I authorize payment of medical benefits to the undersigned physician or supplier for services described below.

SIGNED _____

14. DATE OF CURRENT: ILLNESS (First symptom) OR INJURY (Accident) OR PREGNANCY (LMP)   MM   DD   YY

15. IF PATIENT HAS HAD SAME OR SIMILAR ILLNESS. GIVE FIRST DATE   MM   DD   YY

16. DATES PATIENT UNABLE TO WORK IN CURRENT OCCUPATION   FROM   MM   DD   YY   TO   MM   DD   YY

17. NAME OF REFERRING PHYSICIAN OR OTHER SOURCE

17a. I.D. NUMBER OF REFERRING PHYSICIAN

18. HOSPITALIZATION DATES RELATED TO CURRENT SERVICES   FROM   MM   DD   YY   TO   MM   DD   YY

19. RESERVED FOR LOCAL USE

20. OUTSIDE LAB? $ CHARGES   YES   NO

21. DIAGNOSIS OR NATURE OF ILLNESS OR INJURY. (RELATE ITEMS 1,2,3 OR 4 TO ITEM 24E BY LINE)

1. ___.___   3. ___.___

2. ___.___   4. ___.___

22. MEDICAID RESUBMISSION CODE   ORIGINAL REF. NO.

23. PRIOR AUTHORIZATION NUMBER

24. A. DATE(S) OF SERVICE						B. Place of Service	C. Type of Service	D. PROCEDURES, SERVICES, OR SUPPLIES (Explain Unusual Circumstances) CPT/HCPCS MODIFIER	E. DIAGNOSIS CODE	F. $ CHARGES	G. DAYS OR UNITS	H. EPSDT Family Plan	I. EMG	J. COB	K. RESERVED FOR LOCAL USE
From MM	DD	YY	To MM	DD	YY										

25. FEDERAL TAX I.D. NUMBER   SSN   EIN

26. PATIENT'S ACCOUNT NO.

27. ACCEPT ASSIGNMENT? (For govt. claims, see back)   YES   NO

28. TOTAL CHARGE $

29. AMOUNT PAID $

30. BALANCE DUE $

31. SIGNATURE OF PHYSICIAN OR SUPPLIER INCLUDING DEGREES OR CREDENTIALS (I certify that the statements on the reverse apply to this bill and are made a part thereof.)

SIGNED _____   DATE _____

32. NAME AND ADDRESS OF FACILITY WHERE SERVICES WERE RENDERED (If other than home or office)

33. PHYSICIAN'S, SUPPLIER'S BILLING NAME, ADDRESS, ZIP CODE & PHONE #

PIN#   GRP#

(APPROVED BY AMA COUNCIL ON MEDICAL SERVICE 8/88)   **PLEASE PRINT OR TYPE**

WHCFA-1500-1-90

FORM HCFA-1500   (12-90)
FORM OWCP-1500   FORM RRB-1500

PATIENT AND INSURED INFORMATION

PHYSICIAN OR SUPPLIER INFORMATION

Figure 1-4 *HCFA-1500 Form*

Chapter 1

CHAPTER REVIEW

DEFINE THE TERMS

Write a definition for each term: (Obj. 1-1)

1. Day sheet

    _____

    _____

    _____

2. Patient ledger

    _____

    _____

    _____

3. Superbill

    _____

    _____

    _____

4. CPT-4

    _____

    _____

    _____

5. ICD-9

    _____

    _____

    _____

6. Champus

_____

_____

_____

 CHECK YOUR UNDERSTANDING

7. List five important financial records that are kept by a medical office that processes transactions using a manual system. *(Obj. 1-2)*

Pg 10-11   2+3

_____

_____

_____

_____

8. What is the relationship of the various journals in the medical office to the general ledger? *(Obj. 1-3)*

PG 10 + 11

_____

_____

_____

_____

_____

9. What is the principal responsibility of the medical billing assistant? What are the two main financial records that the medical billing assistant handles when using a manual system? *(Obj. 1-4 and 1-5)*

Pg 11

_____

_____

_____

_____

_____

10. Similar information is found on a day sheet and a patient ledger. What is the difference between these two forms? *(Obj. 1-5)*

PG 13

_____

_____

_____

_____

_____

11. Who in the medical office fills out the superbill? Who uses the information on the superbill and for what purposes? *(Obj. 1-5)*

PG 11

_____

_____

_____

_____

_____

12. What manual tasks does the medical billing assistant perform on a daily basis? *(Obj. 1-5)*

PG 16

_____

_____

_____

_____

13. What tasks does the medical billing assistant perform on a monthly (or other long-term) basis? *(Obj. 1-5)*

PG 16

_____

_____

_____

_____

THINK IT THROUGH

14. From a financial point of view, what is the role and importance of patient billing in the medical office? *(Obj. 1-4)*

Office to run smoothly

_____

_____

_____

_____

_____

_____

_____

_____

_____

_____

Chapter 2

USING THE COMPUTER FOR PATIENT BILLING

WHAT YOU NEED TO KNOW

To complete this chapter, you need to know:

- What the major elements of a medical office accounting system are and how patient billing fits into the system.

- The main responsibilities of a medical billing assistant.

- What financial records the medical billing assistant maintains and what each record contains.

WHAT YOU WILL LEARN

When you finish this chapter, you will be able to:

1. Define the terms used in this chapter.

2. Describe the data files maintained in a medical office database.

3. Define the options available in a computerized patient accounting system.

4. Compare a manual patient billing system with a computerized system.

5. Start and exit *MediSoft*.

6. Make selections from *MediSoft* menus.

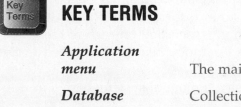

KEY TERMS

Application menu   The main menu for the program. (See *Menu bar*.)

Database   Collection of information (data) arranged logically so that it can be stored and retrieved.

Data file   Subset of data that is part of a larger database. (See *List*.)

Dialog box	A window with data entry fields and other controls that allow a user to interact with a program.
Field	Element of information consisting of one or more characters (letters, numbers, and symbols) displayed on the screen with a descriptive label such as "Today's Date," "Last Name," "Address," "Diagnosis," and so on.
List	Term used by *MediSoft* to refer to a subset of data that is part of a larger database. (See *Data file*.)
Menu	List of options that shows the actions you instruct a program to perform.
Menu bar	The main menu of a program that appears horizontally across the top of an application's window. (See *Application menu*.)
MultiLink code	Code used to identify a group of CPT-4 procedure codes.
Program date	Date used by the *MediSoft* program to process transactions. Unless specifically set, the program uses the current date stored by the computer.
Speed key	A single key that lets you quickly select a menu option. The underlined letter in a menu option identifies its corresponding speed key.
Status bar	Area at the bottom of the screen used to display messages directing you to perform an action or giving you helpful information.
Submenu	Secondary menu reached by making a selection from another menu.
Toolbar	The area just below the application menu that includes buttons used to perform specific functions.
Window	An area on the screen in which a program displays information such as the menu bar, a status bar, a dialog box, or a report.

MEDICAL OFFICE DATABASES ◆

In Chapter 1, you learned that the major documents used or produced in a patient billing system are superbills, day sheets, patient ledgers, patient statements, insurance forms, and patient information forms. Important information is recorded on each of these documents, and information from one document is often used in the preparation of others.

In a typical medical office using a manual system, basic information about each patient's visit is:

1. Recorded first on a superbill.

2. Transferred from a superbill to a day sheet.

3. Posted from a superbill or day sheet to the patient ledger.

4. Included on the patient statement for the month.

5. Used in preparing an insurance form for the visit.

All information collected and recorded on the various documents in an office can be considered part of a medical office database. A **database** is a collection of information (data) arranged logically so that it can be stored and retrieved.

In a medical office such as the one described in Chapter 1, where all records are kept manually, the database consists of paper records kept in files. When a computerized patient billing system such as *MediSoft* is used, the database is maintained by the computer. Printed copies of data are filed in the office as a backup in the event of computer problems.

Table 2-1 on page 28 shows several of the data files included in a *MediSoft* database. Each **data file** is a subset of a medical office's complete database. *MediSoft* also refers to these data files as **lists**. Each data file or list consists of smaller elements called **fields,** as shown in the table.

For example, the *MediSoft* program maintains a **MultiLink code** data file that consists of special codes where one code is used to represent a group of procedures. Typically, these codes are used when several procedures are commonly performed together. A code such as STREP, for example, could be set up to include both a strep culture and a penicillin injection. Some fields in the MultiLink data file or list include the MultiLink code number, description, and procedure code links.

Information stored in a medical office database is used for a variety of purposes. For example, the patient data file is used to update patient ledgers, create patient statements, and prepare insurance forms. When you work with a computerized patient billing system, you may not be aware of how much of the database is being used. The computerized system allows you to retrieve data from and add new data to the database automatically as you work.

OPTIONS IN A COMPUTERIZED PATIENT BILLING SYSTEM ◆

A computerized patient billing system allows you to perform many, if not all, of the tasks performed in a manual system. The **menus** and **submenus** in the *MediSoft* system provide access to the program features needed to maintain a patient accounting system.

DATA FILE/LIST	DESCRIPTION	FIELDS
Practice Information	General information related to a medical practice.	Practice name, address, phone number, practice type, and tax identification number.
Patients/Guarantors	Personal information about each patient and guarantor.	Patient identification code, last name, first name, address, phone number, birth date, gender, age, social security number, assigned provider, and employment.
Cases	Pertinent information about the procedures and transactions related to each patient.	Case number, personal patient information (marital status, student status, employment, etc.), case description, account data (provider, referral source, attorney, billing code, etc.), diagnosis, insurance policy information (insured, relationship to insured, insurance carrier, policy number, etc.), condition, Medicaid/Champus information, and miscellaneous data.
Procedure, Payment, and Adjustment Codes	Codes used to simplify the entry of procedures, payments, and adjustments. For procedures, the CPT-4 codes are used to identify specific procedures performed. Payment codes, for example, could be set up to identify a cash payment by a patient. Another code could be used to identify a payment made by check.	Code number, code type (procedure charge, payment, or adjustment), service type, place of service, and charge amount.
MultiLink Codes	List of codes that allows a medical practice to group multiple procedures codes (CPT-4) into a single code.	MultiLink code number, description, and procedure code links.
Diagnosis Codes	List of standard diagnosis codes based on the ICD-9 codes.	Diagnosis code number, diagnosis description, and alternate codes.
Insurance Carriers	List of insurance companies used by a medical practice to process patient claims.	Insurance carrier code number, address, phone number, contact, plan name, type (government, HMO, PPO, etc.), procedure/diagnosis code information, and electronic claims management information.
Providers	Information related to any staff member (doctor, nurse, therapist, physician's aide, etc.) who performs services for a patient.	Provider code number, name, credentials, address, phone numbers, license number, specialty, personal identification numbers, and other identification codes.
Addresses	List of addresses such as employers, referral sources, attorneys, and medical labs. Usually, patient addresses are not stored in this data file.	Addressee code number, name, address, type (employer, referral source, lab, etc.), fax number, and contact.

Table 2-1 *MediSoft Lists*

MediSoft Application Menu

The application menu in *MediSoft*, shown in Figure 2-1, appears after you start the program. The **application menu** or **menu bar** is the main menu that appears horizontally across the top of an application's window. The **toolbar**, which is a group of buttons used to perform various functions, appears just below the application menu in the main window. A **window** is the area on a screen where the program displays information such as its menu bar, status bar, and program date. A **status bar** shows messages related to the program, and the **program date** is the date *MediSoft* uses to process transactions.

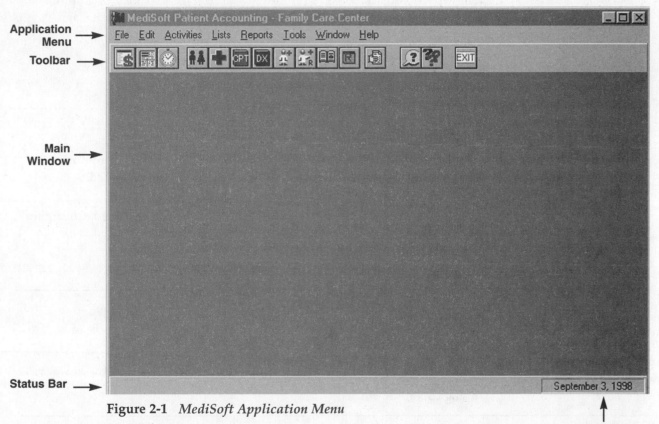

Figure 2-1 *MediSoft Application Menu*

The options shown in the application menu (File, Edit, Activities, Lists, Reports, Tools, Window, and Help) represent the categories of features available in the *MediSoft* program. As a medical billing assistant, you will most likely not use all of these options; some are used by other staff members. The information shown in Table 2-2, pages 30-31, describes most of the options available in the *MediSoft* program and explains which options a medical billing assistant would use.

As presented in Table 2-2, the *MediSoft* program organizes the program options by category. For example, all of the reports are grouped in the Reports menu. To print the Patient Day Sheet report,

OPTIONS	DESCRIPTION	USED IN BILLING?
FILE		
Open Practice	Allows you to open a database file for a medical practice. This option is useful if you are using *MediSoft* for more than one practice.	Only indirectly to open a practice database.
New Practice	Creates a new database for a medical practice.	No, usually others will set up a practice.
Convert Data	Allows you to convert data from earlier versions on *MediSoft*.	No.
Backup Data	Allows you to back up data.	Yes, for making a backup of a medical practice's database.
View Backup Disks	Lets you view data on a backup disk.	Yes.
Restore Data	Restores data from a backup disk.	Yes.
Set Program Date	Changes the date used by *MediSoft* to process data.	Yes.
Practice Information	Allows you to make changes in an existing practice.	No.
Program Options	Set backup parameters, startup options, and data entry conventions.	No, most program options will already be configured.
File Maintenance	Lets you rebuild a medical office database and perform other maintenance options.	Yes, but only if the database files are damaged or need to be purged.
Exit	Quits the program.	Yes.
EDIT		
Undo *Cut* *Copy* *Paste* *Delete*	All of these options provide editing capabilities while you input data. You can undo your last entry in a field, or use the cut/copy/paste options to make processing data more efficient.	Yes, while entering data into the system.
ACTIVITIES		
Enter Transactions	Allows you to record charges to patients for office visits and other procedures. You can enter customer payments, adjustments, and insurance payments.	Yes.
Claim Management	Provides options to print claim forms or send them electronically.	Yes.
Appointment Book	Can be used to schedule patient appointments, repeating appointments, or other activities for each provider.	No, other staff members are usually responsible for scheduling.

Table 2-2 *MediSoft Application Menu Options*

OPTIONS	DESCRIPTION	USED IN BILLING?
LISTS *Patients/Guarantors and Cases* *Patient Recall* *Procedure/Payment/ Adjustment Codes* *MultiLink Codes* *Diagnosis Codes* *Insurance Carriers* *Addresses* *EMC Receivers* *Referring Providers* *Providers* *Billing Codes*	The options in the Lists menu allow you to update all of the data files or lists stored in a medical office's database. For example, you would use the *Patients/ Guarantors and Cases* option to add new patient information or to update an existing patient's information. (See Table 2-1 for a description of these lists.)	Yes.
REPORTS *Patient Day Sheet* *Procedure Day Sheet* *Patient Ledger* *Patient Aging* *Practice Analysis* *Primary Insurance Aging* *Secondary Insurance Aging* *Tertiary Insurance Aging* *Patient Statements* *Custom Report List* *Design Custom Reports and Bills*	Provides access to reports including patient ledgers, day sheets, and procedure day sheets. You can also create your own custom reports and bills.	Yes.
TOOLS *Calculator* *View File* *System Information* *Modem Check*	Provides access to tools such as a calculator, a utility to view the content of a file, and an option to examine information about your computer.	No, except for the calculator if you need to manually calculate a charge.
WINDOW	Allows you to switch between windows (e.g., Patient List and Diagnosis List) used by the program.	Not directly; these options are used for navigation purposes, not billing.
HELP	Provides detailed information about each of *MediSoft's* options. Also, includes information needed to register the program.	Not directly; the options in this menu provide information to help you use the program more efficiently.

Table 2-2 *MediSoft Application Menu Options (Concluded)*

you would pull down the Reports menu and then choose the *Patient Day Sheet* option. Figure 2-2 shows the options in the Reports menu.

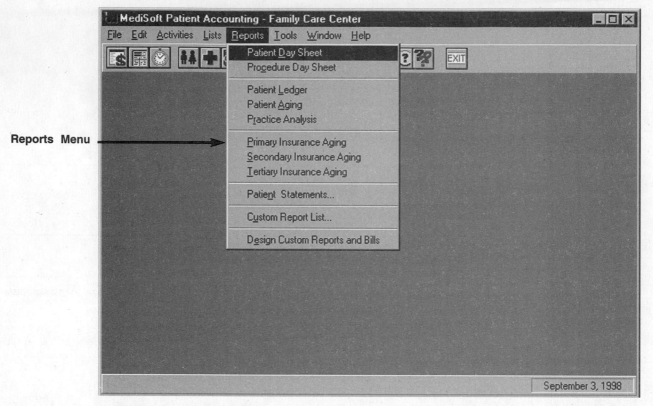

Figure 2-2 *Reports Menu*

Toolbar

The toolbar included as part of the *MediSoft* main window provides an alternative method to access many of the program's options. All of the options in the Activities application menu can be selected from the toolbar. Also, many of the Lists menu options, the *Custom Report List* option, and Help options can be selected by clicking on the corresponding button in the toolbar. Each of the toolbar options are identified in Figure 2-3.

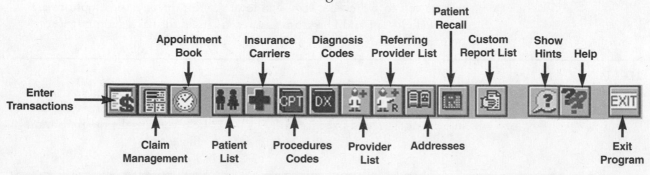

Figure 2-3 *MediSoft Toolbar Options*

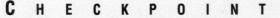

CHECKPOINT

1. A new patient visits the office and is treated for allergies. Which option from the Lists menu would you use to enter the patient and case information?

   P16 + Case option Lists

2. You need to print a day sheet at the end of a day. Which option would you choose to print this report?

   Reports

3. A patient recently changed jobs and is now covered by a health insurance company not listed in the medical office's database. Which option would you choose to add the information for this new health insurance company?

   IC

PRACTICE EXERCISE 2-1

Starting MediSoft

Follow the instructions provided here to start the *MediSoft for Windows* software.

1. Turn on the computer and insert your data disk into Drive A (or B).

   IMPORTANT: Never remove your data disk from the drive while the *MediSoft* program is running. Be sure to quit the program before you remove the data disk.

2. Refer to the appropriate instructions that correspond to your computer system. The program requires a few moments to start and open the practice data from the floppy disk drive.

   Windows 3.1: Locate the *MediSoft* program icon. Double-click the program icon to start the software.

   Windows 95: Click the **Start** button on the Taskbar. Highlight the **Programs** menu and locate the *MediSoft* folder. Select the *MediSoft* option to start the software.

3. Verify that the program opened the Family Care Center Practice data. The program name and current practice information (*i.e., MediSoft — Family Care Center*) appear at the top of the window.

   If this is the first time you are using the *MediSoft* program or the practice information was removed, you may have to create a new practice before you can continue. Follow these steps to create a new practice.

◆ Click the **Create a new set of data** button if prompted, or choose the *New Practice* option from the File menu.

◆ Enter **Family Care Center** for the practice name and **A:\FAMILY** for the data path. (Use **B:\FAMILY** if your data disk is located in Drive B.)

◆ Click the **Create** button.

◆ When prompted that data already exist in this directory, click the **Yes** button to continue. If you don't see this message, you may have entered the wrong path. Indicate that you do not want to continue. Go back and enter the path again.

◆ Review the information in the Practice Information dialog box, and then click the **Save** button to continue. A **dialog box** is a window with data entry fields and other controls that allow a user to interact with a program.

4. Pull down the **File** menu and choose the *Set Program Date* option. (See Figure 2-4.) Enter **September 4, 1998** for the date unless instructed otherwise in the tutorial or simulation. Click the **Check mark** button to complete the data entry. Be sure to enter the date correctly since *MediSoft* relies on the date to process information. You are now ready to begin using the software.

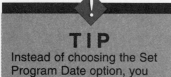

TIP

Instead of choosing the Set Program Date option, you can simply click on the program date shown in the lower, right corner of the window to access this option.

Click here to accept the date.   Use these options to

Click here to cancel the option. →

| | September ▼ | 1998 ▼ |
Sun	Mon	Tue	Wed	Thu	Fri	Sat
30	31	1	2	3	4	5
6	7	8	9	10	11	12
13	14	15	16	17	18	19
20	21	22	23	24	25	26
27	28	29	30	1	2	3
4	5	6	7	8	9	10

Click in this area to set the day.

September 4, 1998

Figure 2-4
Program Date Entry

NAVIGATING THROUGH THE SOFTWARE ━━━━━━━━━━━━━━━◆

If you are familiar with other *Windows* applications such as a word processor or spreadsheet, you should be comfortable using the *MediSoft* program. To choose an option from the application menu, you can use the mouse or the keyboard. Other controls such as buttons, list boxes, input fields, and check boxes let you interact with the program. Follow the steps in Practice Exercise 2-2 to practice choosing options from the application menu.

PRACTICE EXERCISE 2-2

Using the Application Menu

Follow these steps to choose an option from the application menu using a mouse.

1. Position the mouse pointer on the Lists menu and press the primary mouse button once to display the menu options.

2. Move the mouse pointer to highlight the *Diagnosis Codes* option and then click the mouse button again to select the option.
   The Diagnosis List window should appear on your screen. Using the options available in this window, you could add, edit, or delete diagnosis codes for the medical practice.

3. Click the **Close** button shown at the bottom of the Diagnosis List window to close the window.

4. Position the mouse pointer on the **Diagnosis Code List** button in the toolbar and then click the mouse button.
   As you can see, this is another way to select some of the options in the application menu.

5. Close the Diagnosis List window.

6. Click on each of the application menu items to view the available options.

Now, use your keyboard to select a menu option.

1. Press the **ALT** key once to access the menu bar.

2. Use the right arrow key to highlight the Help menu.

3. Press the **ENTER** key to display the Help menu options.

4. Press the down arrow key to highlight the *Getting Started* option and press **ENTER** to select it.
   The Getting Started help information should appear on your screen. Using the controls in this window, you can access all of the other help topics.

5. Press **ALT + F** simultaneously to access the File menu in the Help window. Then press the speed key **X** for the *Exit* option. Choosing **Exit** closes the Help window.

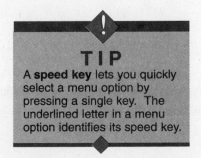

TIP

A **speed key** lets you quickly select a menu option by pressing a single key. The underlined letter in a menu option identifies its speed key.

◆

When you finish using the *MediSoft* program at the end of each day, you need to back up your data and then exit the program. Since you have not made any changes to the Family Care Center database, you do not need to make a backup at this time. The backup feature will be discussed in a later chapter. After you exit the program, remove the data disk from the floppy drive and store it in a safe place.

IMPORTANT: Do not remove the data disk until you completely exit the *MediSoft* program.

PRACTICE EXERCISE 2-3

Exiting the MediSoft Program

To exit the *MediSoft* program:

1. Pull down the **File** menu and choose *Exit*, or click the **Exit** button on the toolbar.

2. When the backup reminder appears, click the **Exit Program** button.

3. Remove your data disk from the disk drive.

COMPARING A COMPUTERIZED BILLING SYSTEM WITH A MANUAL BILLING SYSTEM ◆

As you have learned in this chapter, the *MediSoft* program includes numerous options that can be used by a medical billing assistant to maintain a computerized patient accounting system. A patient accounting program such as *MediSoft* offers many advantages over a manual system. Several advantages of a computerized system are discussed in the following sections.

Reduces Steps to Record Data

One important advantage is that a computerized system eliminates unnecessary steps. For example, *MediSoft* allows you to enter data in one place and then it automatically uses that information in many other areas. Table 2-3, page 37, identifies the steps to transfer information from the superbill to prepare a day sheet and a patient ledger. The steps for a manual system are compared with a computerized system. As you can see, many of the steps required

Manual System	**Computerized System**
Provider fills out a superbill, and a person at the front desk totals the charge and collects payment.	Same.
Medical billing assistant writes the superbill information on a day sheet.	Medical billing assistant enters the case information using the *Patient List* option and then enters the charges with the *Enter Transactions* option.
Medical billing assistant totals columns on a day sheet at the end of a day.	Automatically updated by the program.
Medical billing assistant uses a day sheet at the end of a day to write information on the patient ledgers.	Automatically updated by the program.
Medical billing assistant calculates each patient's new balance.	Automatically calculated by the program.

Table 2-3 *Manual System Versus Computerized System*

in a manual system are performed automatically by a patient accounting program such as *MediSoft*.

Provides Greater Accuracy

Another advantage of a computerized system is that records tend to be more accurate than those generated in a manual system. When you write data manually several times, you may make an error. It is also possible to make errors in calculations. If you are careful to enter data accurately the first time in a computerized system, the data will be accurate each time it is used by the system.

Saves Time by Using Codes

As you enter information into a computerized patient billing system, you do not have to reenter it over and over. The system uses numeric and alphanumeric codes to represent certain kinds of information including the following: patients, procedures, diagnoses, providers, and insurance companies. You could, for example, identify an insurance carrier such as Blue Cross/Blue Shield using the number 4 as the code. Then, when you need to identify a patient's insurance company (e.g., Blue Cross/Blue Shield), you only have to enter or select the appropriate code number. The software matches the code to the corresponding insurance company in the insurance data file.

Chapter

2 | CHAPTER REVIEW

Define Terms

DEFINE THE TERMS

Write a definition for each term: (Obj. 2-1)

1. Database

   _____

   _____

   _____

2. Application menu

   _____

   _____

   _____

3. List

   _____

   _____

   _____

4. Window

   _____

   _____

   _____

5. Field

   _____

   _____

   _____

6. List and describe three of the data files (or lists) that are part of the *MediSoft* database. (*Obj. 2-2*)

   Pg 27

   _____

   _____

   _____

   _____

   _____

   _____

7. What are the options shown in the *MediSoft* application menu? (*Obj. 2-3*)

   Pg 29

   _____

   _____

   _____

   _____

8. Which application menu includes the option to print a day sheet? (*Obj. 2-3*)

   Pg 29 bottom

   _____

   _____

   _____

9. How would you change the *MediSoft* program date to September 8, 1998? (*Obj. 2-3*)

   Pg 34

   _____

   _____

   _____

   _____

   _____

THINK IT THROUGH

10. Describe the advantages of a computerized billing system over a manual patient accounting system. *(Obj. 2-4)*

 (a 3C·37

_____

_____

_____

_____

_____

_____

_____

_____

_____

Chapter 2 ◆ *Using the Computer for Patient Billing*

Chapter 3

MANAGING DATA WITH A COMPUTERIZED SYSTEM

WHAT YOU NEED TO KNOW

To complete this chapter, you need to know:

◆ Options available in a computerized system.

◆ Start-up and exit procedures for *MediSoft*.

◆ Steps to select menu options.

WHAT YOU WILL LEARN

When you finish this chapter, you will be able to:

1. Define the terms used in this chapter.

2. Use the computer keyboard to enter information in *MediSoft*.

3. Navigate the *MediSoft* data entry windows.

4. Search for information in *MediSoft*.

5. Add a new procedure code to a *MediSoft* database.

6. Create a new chart number for a patient.

7. Back up your data.

KEY TERMS

Chart number   A unique number that identifies each patient; in *MediSoft*, used on all documents that pertain to that patient.

Combo box   Special data entry field that allows you to type information or select an item from a list.

Cursor keys   Keys marked with arrows that control movement of the cursor on the screen. Also called *arrow keys*.

| *Folder* | A means to arrange information by categories in a data entry window. |
| *Function keys* | Keys labeled "F1," "F2," and so on; used to perform special functions in software. |

ENTERING DATA

When you work with a computerized patient billing system, you use the keys on a computer keyboard to input information (such as words or numbers) and to select options (such as those that tell the computer to print or save a file). The keyboard that you use is very much like a typewriter keyboard, but it has some important differences.

Keyboard

The keyboard, like a typewriter keyboard, contains letter keys and number keys, which are located above the top row of letters. In addition, there are **cursor keys** (marked with arrows) and **function keys** (labeled "F1," "F2," and so forth), as well as other keys. Often, the keyboard has a separate numeric keypad as well. Some of these keys and their uses are described in Table 3-1, on page 45. A standard and an extended keyboard are shown below in Figure 3-1.

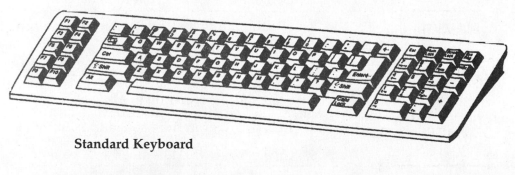

Standard Keyboard

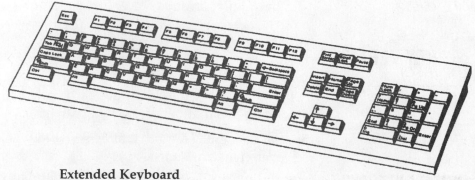

Extended Keyboard

Figure 3-1 *Standard and Extended Keyboards*

KEY	DESCRIPTION
Function keys (F1, F2, and so on)	Most standard keyboards have 10 function keys and extended keyboards usually include 12 function keys. Function keys let you quickly choose an option. For example, you can press F1 to access the Help information.
ENTER	When entering data, press this key to accept the data you key into a field. If a button is selected, you can press ENTER to perform the command associated with that button.
TAB	Press this key to move from one field to another.
Left and right arrow keys	Use the left and right arrow keys to move the cursor (flashing vertical line or block) within an input field. The cursor moves in the direction of the arrow key.
CAPS LOCK	Press this key to toggle the entry mode. If you enable the Caps Lock mode, all letters that you type appear in uppercase without the need to hold down the SHIFT key.
SHIFT	Hold down the SHIFT key while you type a letter to enter an uppercase letter.
NUM LOCK	Press the NUM LOCK key to enable the numeric keys on the ten-key keypad (if available). When the Num Lock indicator is off, you cannot use the keypad to enter numbers.
INSERT (INS)	Press the INSERT key to toggle between two different modes—Insert and Overstrike. In Insert mode, the program "inserts" any characters you type into the input field. If the program is in Overstrike mode, the program "replaces" the currently highlighted character with the character you type.
BACKSPACE	Use the BACKSPACE key to delete the character immediately to the left of the cursor.
DELETE (DEL)	While in Insert mode, press the DELETE key to delete the character to the right of the cursor. If the program is in Overstrike mode, press the DELETE key to delete the currently highlighted character.
ESCAPE (ESC)	Press this key to cancel an operation.
CTRL and ALT	These keys work in combination with other keys to perform special tasks. If a window includes a "New" button, for example, you can hold down the ALT key and type the letter N to select that button rather than clicking it with a mouse.

Table 3-1 *Keyboard Layout*

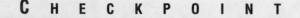

CHECKPOINT

1. Which key would you press to change the entry mode so that you can type over existing text in an input field?

   ENTER or TAB

2. Which key would you use to delete a character to the left of the cursor?

   Backspace key

Moving Around in a Data Entry Window

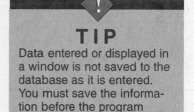

TIP

Data entered or displayed in a window is not saved to the database as it is entered. You must save the information before the program stores it in the database.

To move from field to field in a data entry window or dialog box, press the ENTER key or the TAB key. Or, you can use the mouse to select a field by clicking in it. To move to the previous field, press SHIFT + TAB. If you change the data in a field, pressing ENTER or TAB accepts the new data and then moves to the next field.

Pressing TAB also moves among buttons and other controls in a window. When a button is highlighted or in focus, you can press ENTER to select it. With the mouse, you can simply click a button to perform the associated action.

CHECKPOINT

3. Which key would you press to move from a name field to an address field in a patient information window?

   ENTER or TAB

4. Does the *MediSoft* program automatically store data in its database when you enter data in a field and press the TAB key?

   No

Selecting Information from a List

The *MediSoft* program simplifies the process of entering certain kinds of data by presenting you with a list of items to choose from. For example, when a data entry window requires that you enter a patient code, you can type the code or you can select the code number from a list. This special data entry field is called a combo box. A **combo box** provides space for you to enter data, and it also includes a small button with an arrow (black triangle) at the right edge of the field. (See the *Chart* and *Case* fields in Figure 3-2, page 49.)

Using your mouse, you click on the Arrow button in a combo box to display a list of choices. Then, click on an item in the list to choose it. Use the scroll bar to view the contents of the pop-up list. To close the list without selecting an item, click the Arrow button again.

You can also select an item from a combo box list using your keyboard. First, move to the field by pressing the TAB key. Then, press the down arrow key to display the list of choices. Use the up/down arrow keys, PAGE UP, PAGE DOWN, HOME, or END to move through the list. To select an item, highlight it and then press ENTER.

Correcting Text

What if you misspell a patient's name while entering it in a data entry field? Is it necessary to erase the entire field and start over? If you make a mistake entering text in a field, you can correct it by using the following keys to position the cursor anywhere in a field. If necessary, use the BACKSPACE and DELETE keys to delete any incorrect text. Then, enter the correct information.

KEY		ACTION
Left Arrow	←	Press the left arrow key to move the cursor one character to the left.
Right Arrow	→	Press the right arrow key to move the cursor one character to the right.
Home	Home	Press the HOME key to position the cursor at the beginning of a data entry field.
End	End	Press the END key to position the cursor at the end of the text in a field.

Table 3-2 *Keys Used in Text Correction*

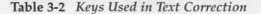

PRACTICE EXERCISE 3-1

Entering and Editing Data

Follow these steps to practice entering information and correcting errors.

1. Start the *MediSoft* program. (Refer to the instructions on page 33.)

2. Set the program date to September 4, 1998.

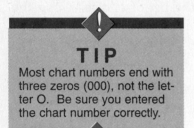

3. Pull down the **Activities** menu and select the *Enter Transactions* option. Or, click the **Enter Transactions** button on the toolbar. An empty Transaction Entry window appears as shown in Figure 3-2, page 49.

4. Type **BELHE000** in the *Chart* field and press **ENTER**.

5. Make sure that **2** (Physical Exam) is entered in the *Case* field. If not, enter the case number now.

> **TIP**
> Most chart numbers end with three zeros (000), not the letter O. Be sure you entered the chart number correctly.

6. Click the **New** button to enter a new transaction.

7. Click the **Payment** tab in the Transaction Entry window or press the speed key **ALT + P** to access the *Payment* folder. The folder tabs do not appear until after you click the button to begin a new transaction.

The *MediSoft* program often arranges information in a window by different categories. (See Figure 3-3.) For example, the Transaction Entry window includes three areas or folders (*Charge*, *Payment*, and *Adjustment*) associated with a patient transaction. You can access any of these folders by clicking on the tab at the top of the folder or by using the corresponding speed key.

8. In the *Dates-From* field, enter the date **September 2, 1998**. To enter the date using the keyboard, type **9/2/98** or **090298** and press **ENTER**.

9. Now change the date back to **September 4, 1998**. This time use the mouse to click on the small **Calendar** button next to the date field. Then set the date accordingly.

> **TIP**
> Remember to press the TAB or Enter key to move to the next field. If you need to go back to a field, press SHIFT+TAB.

10. In the *Pay Code* field, enter **01** to record a cash payment by a patient. Type the code or select it from the list.

11. Enter **Bell, Herbert** in the *Who Paid* field.

12. Move to the *Description* field and type **cash payment**.

13. Type **155.00** in the *Amount* field, but do not press ENTER.

14. Change the amount to **150.00**. Use the arrow keys to move the cursor and then correct the amount.

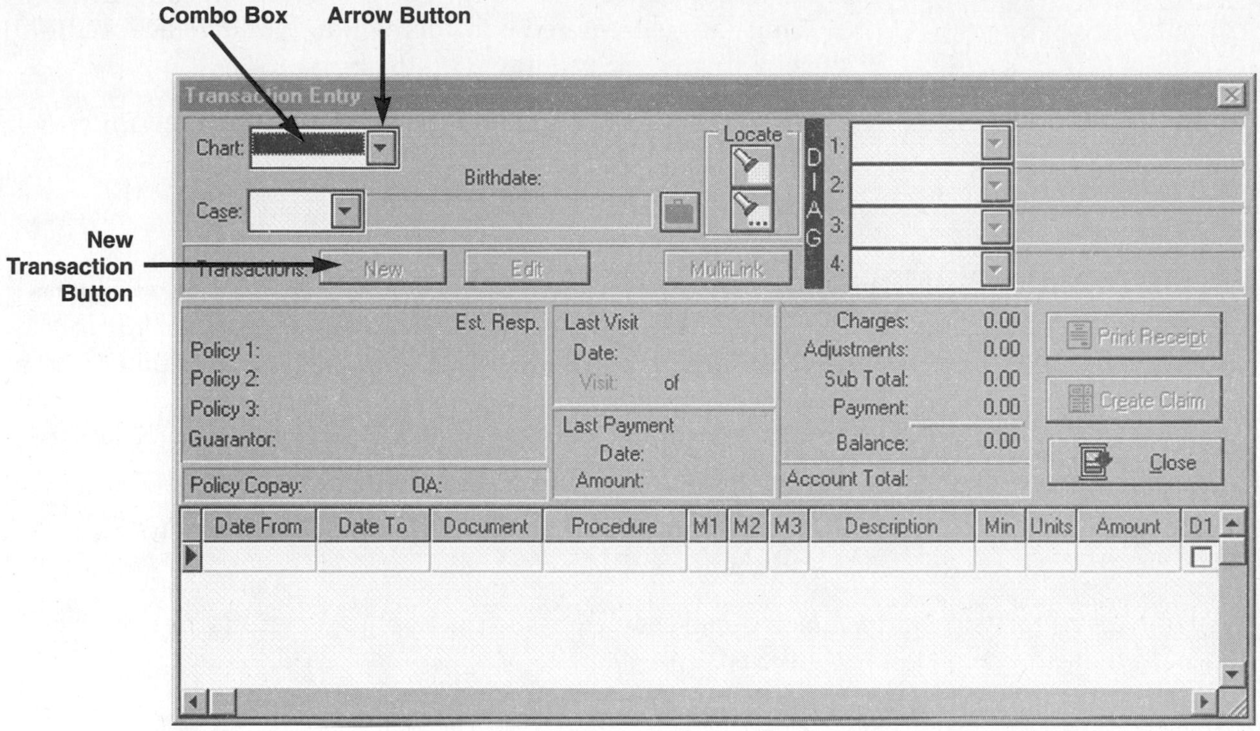

Combo Box   **Arrow Button**

Figure 3-2 *Transaction Entry Window*

Payment Folder Tab   **Adjustment Folder Tab**   **Cancel**

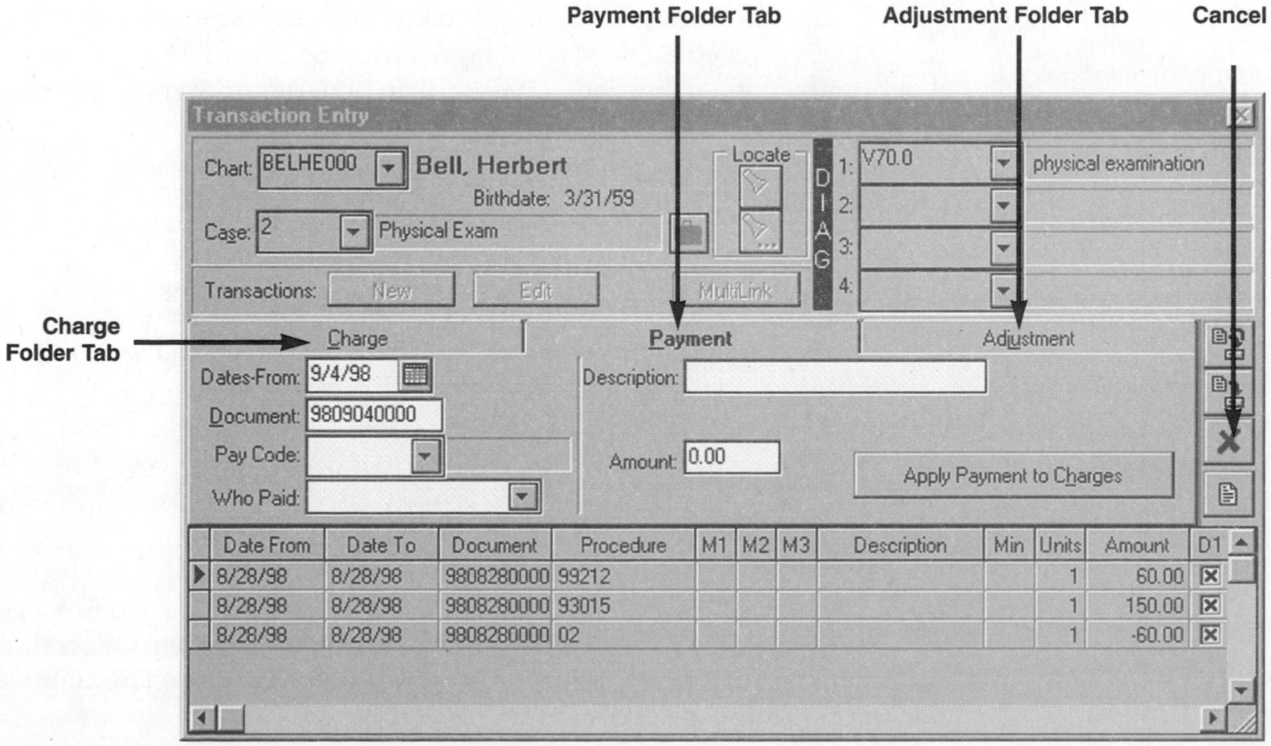

Figure 3-3 *New Transaction Entry Window*

Chapter 3 ◆ *Managing Data with a Computerized System*

15. Click the **Cancel** button so that you do not record any of the data you just entered. In this window, the Cancel button is shown only with a large **X** on the button.

16. Click the **Close** button to close the Transaction Entry window.

PATIENT CHART NUMBERS

The most important patient information is the chart number (sometimes called an *account number*). A **chart number** is a unique number that identifies a patient. *MediSoft* requires that you assign an eight-character chart number to each patient.

◆ A chart number can include any combination of letters (A-Z) and numbers (0-9).

◆ No special characters such as hyphens, periods, or spaces are allowed.

◆ No two chart numbers in the system can be the same.

Medical practices typically use one of two systems for assigning chart numbers as described here, but *MediSoft* will automatically assign a chart number using the first system. You can, however, manually assign any chart number you want.

The first system used by many medical practices and the *MediSoft* program does not require any special coding for the chart number, whether or not a patient is the guarantor (person or party responsible for payment). With this system, bills are mailed to each patient, regardless of whether that person is the guarantor. Here is how the assignment of a chart number in this first system works:

◆ **First three characters:** first three letters of a patient's last name.

◆ **Next two characters:** first two letters of a patient's first name.

◆ **Last three characters:** 000.

If a new chart number generated by the program matches the first five characters of an existing patient chart number, the program uses 001 for the last three characters and so on until it finds an available chart number.

The second system assumes that the guarantor (sometimes referred to as the head of household) should receive the bills for all members of a family. Here is how the assignment of a chart number works in this second system:

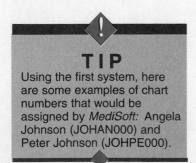

TIP
Using the first system, here are some examples of chart numbers that would be assigned by *MediSoft:* Angela Johnson (JOHAN000) and Peter Johnson (JOHPE000).

TIP

With the system that identifies the guarantor, here are some examples of chart numbers that you could manually assign: James Burke, guarantor (BURKEJA0); Kathryn Burke, daughter (BURKEJA1); and Chad Burke, son (BURKEJA2).

◆ The chart number for all members of the same household must have the same first seven characters.

◆ The guarantor's chart number must end with a 0 (zero).

◆ Chart numbers for other members of a household must end with the digits 1-9.

As with the first system, you may have to make adjustments if there are any conflicts with existing codes.

C H E C K P O I N T

Using the first method described for assigning chart numbers, identify the chart numbers that the *MediSoft* program would generate for these names.

5. William Jackson

JACWI000

6. Julia Hickson

HICJU000

7. Kim Hwang

HWAKI000

SEARCHING IN MEDISOFT

As you work with the software, you may need to locate information stored in a *MediSoft* database. A computer search allows you to find data that match what you have entered, even if you enter only part of the item. Although you may not need to use this feature very often as you work through this tutorial and simulation, the search feature is especially useful when working with a large database. Some medical practices, for example, have thousands of patients. Using the *MediSoft* search feature, you can search for such things as:

◆ Patient chart numbers

◆ Insurance carrier codes

◆ Diagnosis codes

◆ Procedure codes

◆ Addresses

Searching for Patients

The search function works differently depending on the context in which you are searching for data, but the same basic guidelines apply. To begin searching for a patient, you can type the first letter of a patient's last name. As shown in Figure 3-4 below, typing an *F* in the *Search* field locates the first chart number that begins with this letter. In our example, the program points to chart number FELST000 (Feldman, Stanley).

As you type additional characters in the *Search* field, the program will automatically try to match what you type with the information stored in its database. Using this technique, you can focus your search even if you don't know a patient's complete name.

The *MediSoft* program lets you search for patients using any of the following criteria: chart number, last name, secondary identification code, and provider. To change the search criteria, use the *Sort by* combo box. This setting controls the sort order and the search criteria.

TIP

Since chart numbers usually begin with the first three letters of a patient's last name, you can use this information to help you quickly locate a patient's chart number.

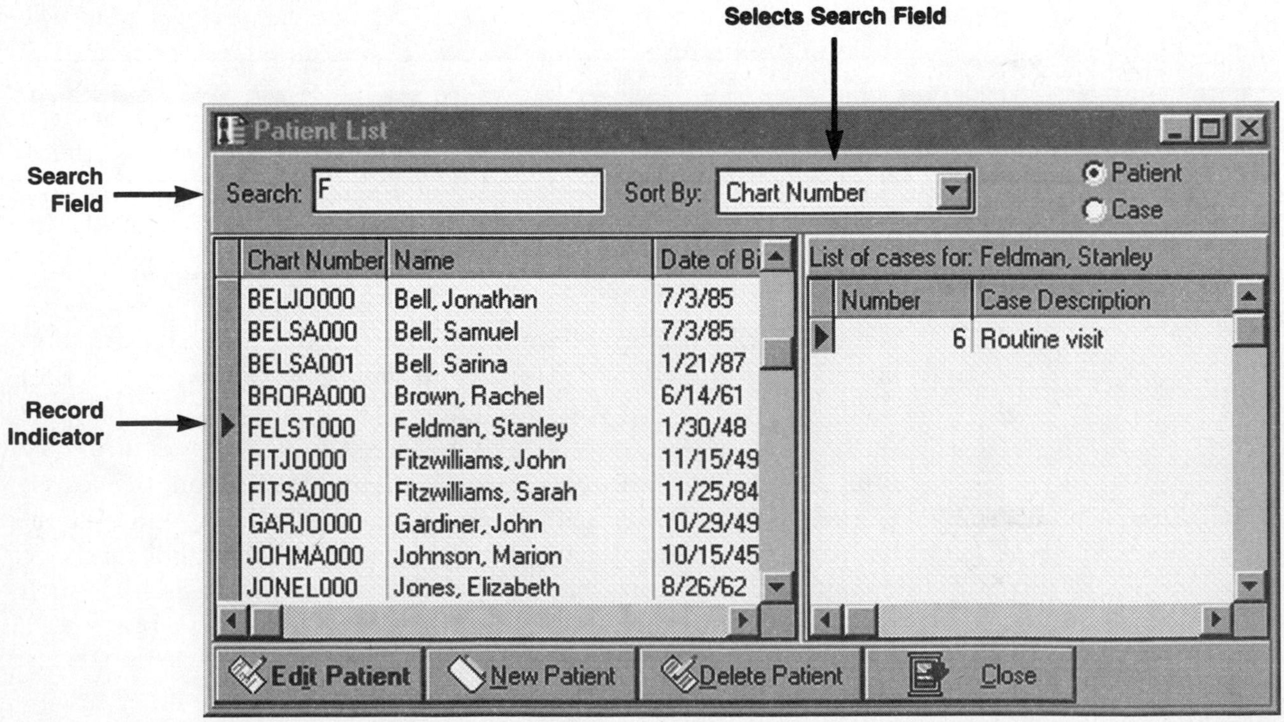

Figure 3-4 *Patient List*

Searching for Other Data

The *MediSoft* program provides the capability to search for data in almost all of its data entry windows. Whether you need to look up a procedure code that begins with *912* or find a diagnosis code, you can use the search feature to help you locate the information you need. Just enter the information you want to find in a *Search* field.

Searching for data is not limited to finding information by entering your search criteria in a *Search* field. The techniques you learned also apply to locating and entering data in a combo box. As you begin typing characters in a combo box, the program will display the closest match. Then, you can use the arrow keys or your mouse to continue searching in the pop-up list.

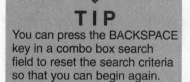

**PRACTICE
EXERCISE 3-2**

Searching for a Patient Chart Number

Practice searching for a patient chart number following these steps:

1. Pull down the **Activities** menu and choose *Enter Transactions*. Or, click the **Enter Transaction** toolbar button.

2. Type the letter **F** in the *Chart* field to begin your search for Sarah Fitzwilliams' chart number.

   The program displays a list of patient chart numbers and highlights the first record that begins with the letter *F* (FELST000—Feldman, Stanley).

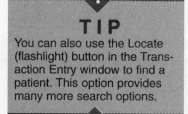

TIP

You can press the BACKSPACE key in a combo box search field to reset the search criteria so that you can begin again.

3. Continue to narrow your search by typing the letter **I** in the field.

   As you can see, the program highlights the first patient chart number that begins with the letters *FI*. You could continue to use this method until you find an exact match or you can select the record once you see it in the list.

4. Use the down arrow key to highlight Sarah's chart number and then press **ENTER**, or use your mouse to select her chart number.

5. Move back to the *Chart* field and then press the **BACKSPACE** key to delete the chart number.

TIP

You can also use the Locate (flashlight) button in the Transaction Entry window to find a patient. This option provides many more search options.

6. Use the steps you just practiced to search for and select Hal Sampson's chart number.

7. Practice finding other chart numbers.

8. Click the **Close** button in the Transaction Entry window when you are finished. Do not save any changes you might have made.

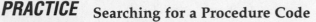

PRACTICE
EXERCISE
3-3

Searching for a Procedure Code

Practice searching for a procedure code following these steps:

1. Pull down the **Lists** menu and choose the *Procedure/ Payment/ Adjustment Codes* option. You can also click the **Procedure Codes** button on the toolbar.

   Suppose you want to find the procedure code for a routine exam for an existing (established) patient, but you can only remember that the code begins with *99*.

2. Enter **99** in the *Search* field as shown in Figure 3-5. The program automatically scrolls the list of procedure codes and points to the first code that begins with the search criteria you entered.

3. Tab twice and the first item beginning with 99 will be highlighted.

4. Use the arrow keys or click on the scroll bar with the mouse to scan the list of procedure codes. Did you find code 99214?

5. Find the code for an ankle X ray. The code begins with *73*.

6. Click the **Close** button to close the window.

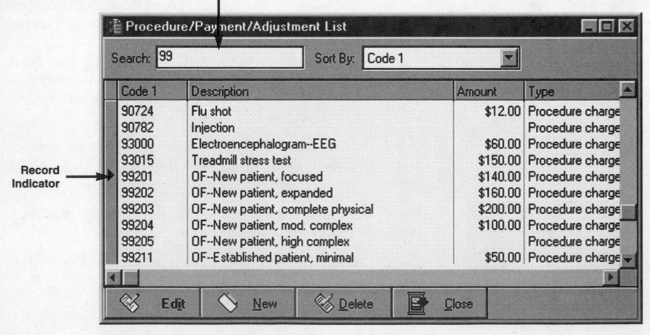

Figure 3-5 *Procedures/Payment/Adjustment List Window*

ADDING NEW CODES ————————————————————◆

When *MediSoft* is set up in an office, not all procedure and diagnosis codes are included in the data files because this would make the files too large and difficult to search. Only the most commonly used codes in a particular office are included. On occasion, however, you may need to add an additional diagnosis, procedure, or other code to the system.

When you add a new code, the information you must enter depends on the code itself. To add a new procedure code, for example, you must complete the following fields: *Code 1*, *Description*, *Code Type*, *Type of Service*, *Place of Service*, *Procedure Code*, and *Charge*. When you add a new diagnosis code, only a *Code* and *Description* field must be completed.

A variety of codes are routinely used in medical office databases to simplify the data entry process and to standardize the information reported to insurance carriers. Often, you will use one or more codes when you set up other codes such as a procedure code. When you set up a new procedure code, you must enter the service type and the place where the service was rendered. The HCFA insurance form, for example, provides a space for you to identify the place of service. The standard Type of Service codes and Place of Service codes are shown in Table 3-3 (below) and Table 3-4 (at the top of page 56). Most insurance carriers accept these codes.

CODE	SERVICE TYPE
1	Medical Care
2	Surgery
3	Consultation
4	Diagnostic X ray
5	Diagnostic Lab
6	Radiation Therapy
7	Anesthesia
8	Surgical Assistance
9	Other Medical
0	Blood Charges

Table 3-3
Type of Service Codes

CODE	PLACE
11	Office
12	Home
21	Inpatient–Hospital
22	Outpatient–Hospital
23	Emergency Room–Hospital
24	Ambulatory Surgical Center

Table 3-4
Place of Service Codes

PRACTICE EXERCISE 3-4

Adding a New Procedure Code

Practice adding a new procedure code by following the steps listed below:

1. Choose *Procedure/Payment/Adjustment Codes* from the Lists menu or use the toolbar to select this option.

2. When the Procedure/Payment/Adjustment List window appears, click the **New** button to add a new procedure code.

3. Enter **99402** in the *Code 1* field.

4. Enter **Counseling, limited** in the *Description* field.

5. In the *Code Type* field, choose **Procedure charge** if it is not already set.

6. Enter **1** for the type of service. (See Table 3-3.)

7. Enter **11** in the *Place of Service* field. (See Table 3-4.)
   Completing the other fields is optional. The *Account Code* field, for example, can be used in combination with a medical office's accounting system. *The Time To Do Procedure* field lets a provider include the number of minutes usually required to perform a procedure.

8. Review the information you entered. If you notice an error, move to the corresponding field to correct the error. (See Figure 3-6.)

9. Click on the *Amounts* folder tab or press **ALT + A**.

10. Enter **50.00** for the charge amount.

11. Click the **Save** button to record the information you entered.

12. Check the list of procedures to make sure that the new code is included.

13. Close the Procedure/Payment/Adjustment List window.

> **TIP**
> Whenever you are instructed to "enter" data, type the information given and then press ENTER or TAB to move to the next field. Remember that pressing SHIFT+TAB moves back to the previous field.

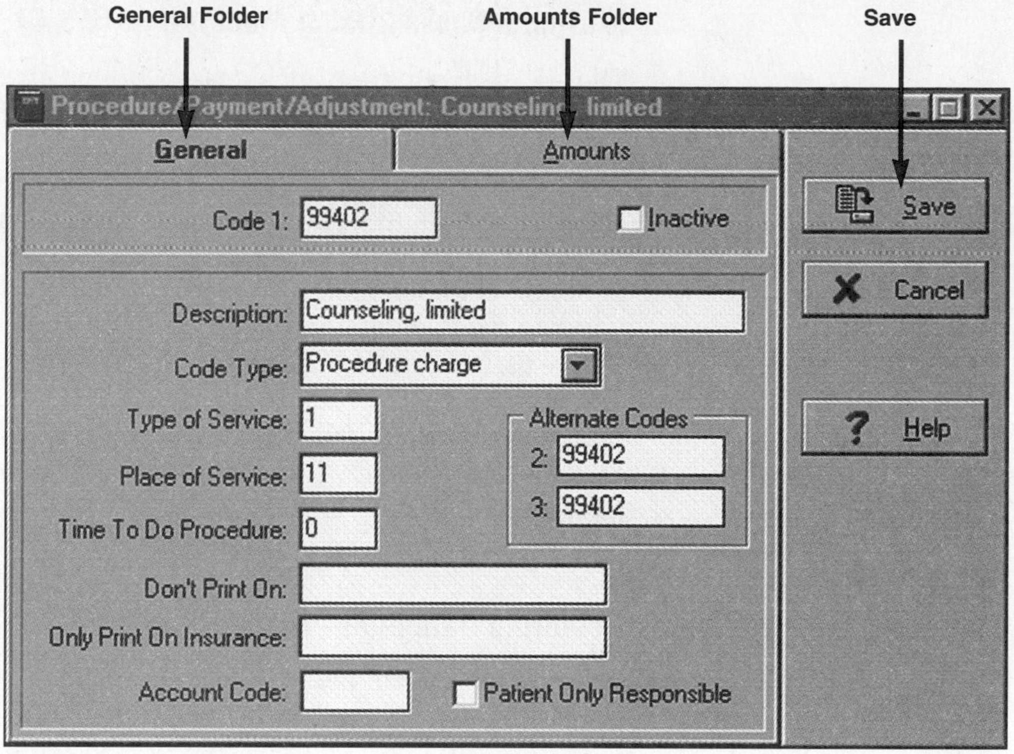

General Folder   Amounts Folder   Save

Figure 3-6 *Completed Procedure Code Entry*

BACKING UP DATA FILES

In an office environment, you should back up the *MediSoft* data on a regular schedule, perhaps on a daily basis using a different disk for each day of the week. You can back up your data to floppy disks, tape, or other media formats. If you use floppy disks, make sure that you have enough formatted disks on hand before you begin the backup process since you cannot interrupt the program to format a disk. Usually, an actual *MediSoft* database will require more than one floppy disk for backup purposes.

> **IMPORTANT:** The information provided below explains how to use the options built into the *MediSoft* program to back up a database, restore data, and view a backup file. Do **NOT** use these options as you work with the software. Since all of your data fit on one disk, you can simply make a copy of your disk to create a backup. If your data are damaged or become unusable, you can use your backup disk. Refer to the instructions on page 5 of the Introduction section if you need help making a copy of a disk.

Chapter 3 ◆ *Managing Data with a Computerized System*

Making a Backup Using MediSoft

The *MediSoft* program includes an option in the File menu that lets you back up your data for a medical office database. *MediSoft* also displays a reminder and gives you the opportunity to make a backup every time you exit the program. Whether you choose the backup option from the menu or select the option to make a backup when you exit, the same *MediSoft* Backup window appears.

When you initiate the backup process, you must choose the source path or location of your data files. You must also identify the destination and the backup filename. Once you start the backup process, the program compresses all of the separate data files into a single backup file and then copies this file to the destination disk or tape.

Restoring Data Files

Chances are you will rarely have a problem that is serious enough to require that you restore data from your backup disk. If you do need to restore data from a backup disk, the program will completely restore (replace) the medical office data files on your hard drive with the data stored in the backup file. You will probably need to reenter all transactions, appointments, and patient data entered since the backup was made.

Viewing Backup Data Files

Sometimes you need to see what is actually on a backup disk to answer questions such as the following:

◆   Is this disk the most recent backup?

◆   Was the backup process performed today?

◆   Did the backup run correctly?

If the disk you are relying on for backup actually has older data than you want or is defective, it won't do you any good. The *View Backup Disks* option in the File menu lets you see when the backup file was created, the original data path, and how many data files are included in the backup file. This option also lists some important statistics for each data file such as actual size, compressed size, and percent compressed.

PRACTICE EXERCISE 3-5

Exiting the Program and Making a Backup Disk

Practice quitting the software and making a backup disk by following these steps:

1. Choose *Exit* from the File menu or use the toolbar to select this option.

2. Click the **Exit Program** button in the Backup Reminder window. Do **NOT** choose the backup option.

3. Make a backup copy of your working disk using the *Windows* operating system utilities, not the *MediSoft* option. Follow the instructions on pages 5-6 of the Introduction if you need help making a backup copy using *Windows 3.1* or *Windows 95*.

4. Store your disks in a safe place.

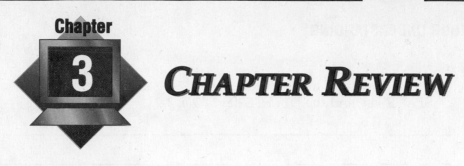

CHAPTER REVIEW

DEFINE THE TERMS

Write a definition for each term: (Obj. 3-1)

1. Combo box

   pg. 47

   _____

   _____

   _____

   _____

2. Chart number

   pg. 50

   _____

   _____

   _____

   _____

3. Function keys

   pg. 44, 45

   _____

   _____

   _____

   _____

4. Folder

   pg. 44

   _____

   _____

   _____

   _____

5. When you enter and edit text, what is the difference between the BACK-SPACE key and the DELETE key? *(Obj. 3-2)*

Pg 45

6. How do you move from one field to another in a *MediSoft* data entry window? How do you move to a previous field? *(Obj. 3-3)*

Pg 46

7. What chart numbers would you create for these patients—John Jackson, Wilma Smith, and David Wong—when it is not important to identify the guarantor or head of household? *(Obj. 3-6)*

Pg 50

8. What capabilities does *MediSoft* provide to search for a patient name or other information stored in a database? *(Obj. 3-4)*

Pg 52

9. Why are codes used in a medical billing program such as *MediSoft*? *(Obj. 3-5)*

Pg 55

10. Explain the steps to add a new procedure code. *(Obj. 3-5)*

Pg 55

11. What options are available in the *MediSoft* program to facilitate the backup process in a medical office? Should you use these features when you make a backup copy of your data? *(Obj. 3-7)*

Pg 57, 58

THINK IT THROUGH

12. You are working in an office entering data from Tuesday when a power failure occurs. When power is restored, you find that much of the data in the *MediSoft* system has errors caused by the failure. What should you do? (*Obj. 3-7*)

_____

_____

_____

_____

_____

_____

_____

_____

_____

_____

_____

_____

_____

ENTERING PATIENT AND CASE INFORMATION

WHAT YOU NEED TO KNOW

To complete this chapter, you need to know how to:

◆ Use the computer keyboard to enter information in *MediSoft*.

◆ Navigate the *MediSoft* software.

◆ Search for information in a *MediSoft* database.

WHAT YOU WILL LEARN

When you finish this chapter, you will be able to:

1. Define the terms used in this chapter.

2. Explain the information requirements for a new patient record.

3. Add a new patient account.

4. Describe the information needs for a new patient case record.

5. Enter a new patient case record.

6. Revise patient information.

7. Explain how to delete a patient account.

KEY TERMS

Billing code	Code used to group or organize patients for billing purposes.
Capitated plan	Type of insurance that pays providers a fixed amount for each patient regardless of the actual medical services rendered.
Co-payment	Standard fee set up by an insurance carrier that is paid to the provider by a patient for medical services rendered.
EMC	Electronic Media Claims—a process for submitting patient claim information directly from one computer to another.

EPSDT	A well-baby program sponsored by Medicaid.
Established patient	A patient who has received medical care from the provider in the last three years.
New patient	A patient who has never visited the medical office or has not received professional care from the provider in the last three years.
Patient information form	Form completed by a patient that includes personal information such as name, address, employer, insurance company, and any known allergies.
Secondary Patient ID	A secondary identification code assigned to a patient. The code can be displayed in lieu of a chart number on certain reports.
Signature on file	Database field that you can use to indicate whether a patient's signature is on file.
Type	Field used to identify an individual or another party as a patient or a guarantor.

HOW PATIENT INFORMATION IS ORGANIZED

As you already learned, the *MediSoft* program requires that you maintain an up-to-date patient list so that the software can process the billing information efficiently. To keep the patient list current, you will need to add information for new patients and update existing patient records. For medical billing purposes, a **new patient** is a patient who has never visited the office or a person who has not seen his/her provider in the past three years. An **established patient** is someone who has received medical care in the office during the past three years.

When a new patient visits a medical office, he/she must fill out a patient information form similar to the one shown in Figure 4-1. The **patient information form** is used to gather personal information such as the patient's name, address, employer, insurance company, and any known allergies. Every new patient must complete one of these forms on his/her initial visit. An established patient may also need to complete this form if any pertinent information such as employer, insurance carrier, or address needs to be updated.

As you can see by looking at Figure 4-1, the patient information form contains a substantial amount of information. Some of this information is used when you add a new patient to the patient/guarantor list. The other information contained on the form is required when you set up a new case for a patient. You will learn how to perform both of these functions in this chapter.

Family Care Center
Patient Information Form

PERSONAL

Name (last, first): _____ Sex: ❑ Male

Address: _____ ❑ Female

_____

Phone No.: (___) _____ Marital Status: ❑ Married ❑ Single

(___) _____ ❑ Separated ❑ Divorced

❑ Widowed

Birth Date: _____

Social Security No.: _____ Student Status: ❑ Full Time ❑ Non-Student

❑ Part Time

EMPLOYMENT

Employer: _____ Employed: ❑ Full Time

Address: _____ ❑ Part Time

_____ ❑ Not Employed

❑ Retired

Phone No.: (___) _____ Ext.: _____ Date: _____

INSURANCE

Primary

Insurance Carrier: _____ Co-Pay Amount: _____

Policy No.: _____ Group No.: _____ Percent Covered: _____

Insured: _____

Relationship
to Insured: ❑ Self ❑ Spouse ❑ Child ❑ Other

Secondary

Insurance Carrier: _____ Co-Pay Amount: _____

Policy No.: _____ Group No.: _____ Percent Covered: _____

Insured: _____

Relationship
to Insured: ❑ Self ❑ Spouse ❑ Child ❑ Other

OTHER

Reason for Visit: _____

Known Allergies: _____

Did another physician refer you to our office? ❑ Yes ❑ No **If yes, who?** _____

Condition Related to: ❑ Auto Accident ❑ Employment Accident ❑ Other Accident

Date Accident Occurred: _____ State Where Accident Occurred: _____

For office use only:

Chart No.: _____ Assigned Provider: _____ Billing Code: _____

Signature on File: ❑ Yes ❑ No

Figure 4-1 *Patient Information Form*

Patient/Guarantor Information Requirements

All of the information you need to enter in a new patient record is provided on a patient information form. Use this information to complete the Patient/Guarantor (new) data entry window shown in Figure 4-2. The option to add a new patient is available in the Patient List window that appears when you choose *Patients/ Guarantors and Cases* from the Lists menu.

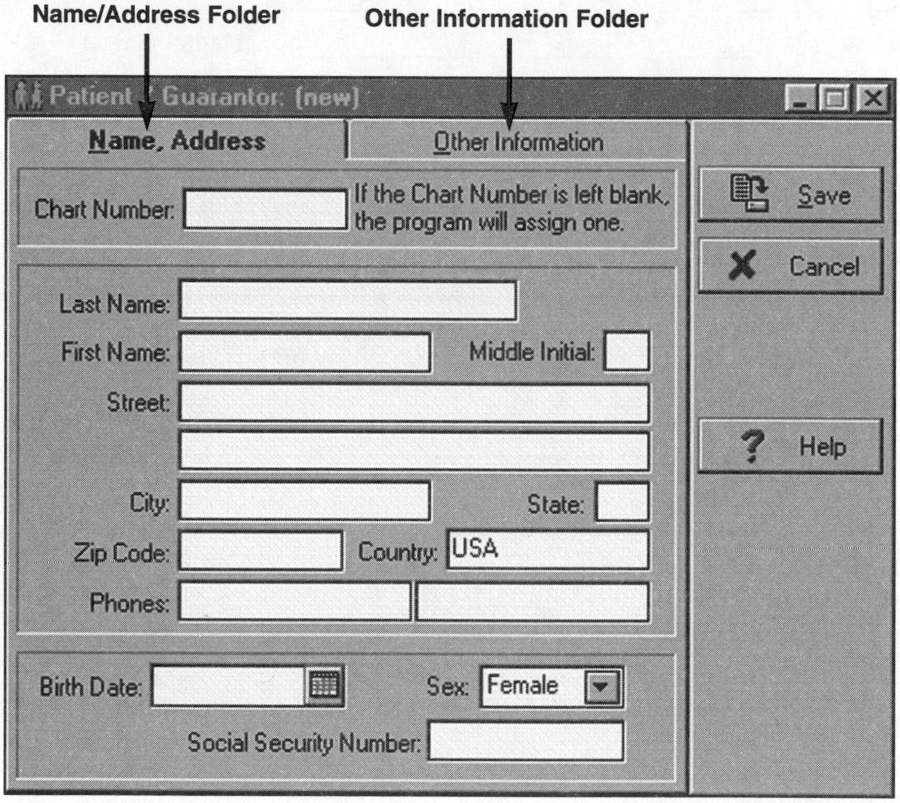

Name/Address Folder   **Other Information Folder**

Figure 4-2 *Patient/Guarantor (New) Window*

To add a new patient, you must enter the following information into the *Name/Address* folder and the *Other Information* folder:

Name/Address Folder

◆ Chart Number

◆ Patient Name (Last Name, First Name, and Initial)

◆ Address (Street, City, State, ZIP Code, and Country)

◆ Home Phone Numbers

◆ Birth Date

◆ Sex

◆ Social Security Number

Other Information Folder

- Type

- Signature on File

- Assigned Provider

- Secondary Patient ID

- Employment (Employer, Status, Work Phone, Location, and Retirement Date)

Most of the information is self-explanatory except for a few of the fields. The **Signature on File** field lets you indicate whether a patient's signature is on file in the office. If a patient's signature is on file, the medical office staff may not have to obtain a signature each time one is needed to complete an insurance claim form, release form, and so on.

The **Type** field is used to identify whether an individual or another party is a patient or a guarantor. In most cases, you will probably use "patient" for the type. However, there may be instances when the information you need to record is not for a patient. Suppose, for example, that you need to add a new patient account for Mary Lopez. She is a student who attends college in a city near the medical office, but her parents live in another state. Mary, however, is still covered by her mother's insurance. In this instance, you would need to set the type to "patient" for Mary and create another record for her mother using "guarantor" as the type. Later, when you enter the case information for Mary, you would reference her mother as the guarantor.

One of the optional fields in a patient/guarantor record is the **Secondary Patient ID** field. This field can serve as a secondary identification code assigned to a patient or guarantor. The code can be displayed in lieu of a chart number on certain reports.

Case Information Requirements

In addition to the patient list information described in the previous section, *MediSoft* stores some patient information such as marital status, account data, diagnosis, insurance policy numbers, and condition in case records. The patient case data is organized into nine different folders. (See Figure 4-3, page 70.) Depending on a medical office's data requirements, a practice may not use all of the fields provided.

Using the data provided on the patient information form, you can complete most of the case fields except for those fields included in the *Diagnosis*, *Medicaid/Champus*, and *Miscellaneous* folders. Later, after the provider completes the patient's superbill, you can use it to enter the additional information.

An overview of the information needed to complete a patient case record is provided in the following paragraphs. Review this information before you continue with the practice exercises.

Case Folders {

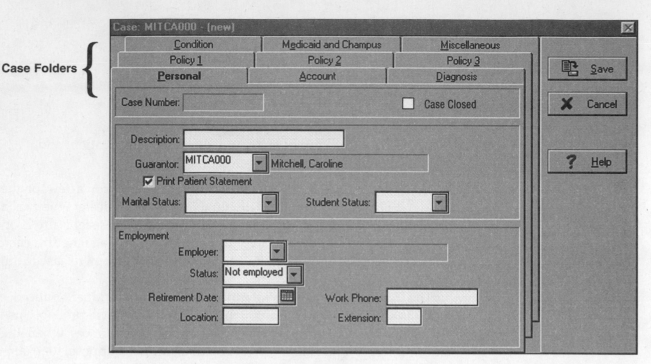

Figure 4-3 *Case Window (Personal Folder)*

Personal   The *Personal* folder contains personal data about a patient along with the case number, which is assigned automatically. When you complete this folder, you must enter a brief case description or reason for the visit. This folder also includes fields to enter the guarantor, marital status, student status, and employment information.

Account   The *Account* folder, as shown in Figure 4-4, page 71, holds pertinent information concerning the patient's account. Use this folder to record the assigned provider, referring provider, referral source, attorney, and facility codes. The codes needed to complete these fields must be set up in the Address file first.

The **billing code**, which is included in the *Account* folder, lets you group or organize patients for billing purposes. How you use this code depends on a medical office's specific billing requirements. For example, you could assign billing code *A* to patients who will receive their bills on the 15th of the month and code *B* for patients billed on the 30th.

Another part of the *Account* folder contains the visit series information. Some insurance companies may require that the patient receive authorization before seeking medical services. A carrier may also authorize only a specific number of visits. In these instances, you can use this area to record the necessary information.

Diagnosis   After a provider completes a patient's superbill, you can use it to enter the diagnosis information in the *Diagnosis* folder. You may enter up to four different diagnosis codes. As you may recall, these codes are stored in the Diagnosis data file.

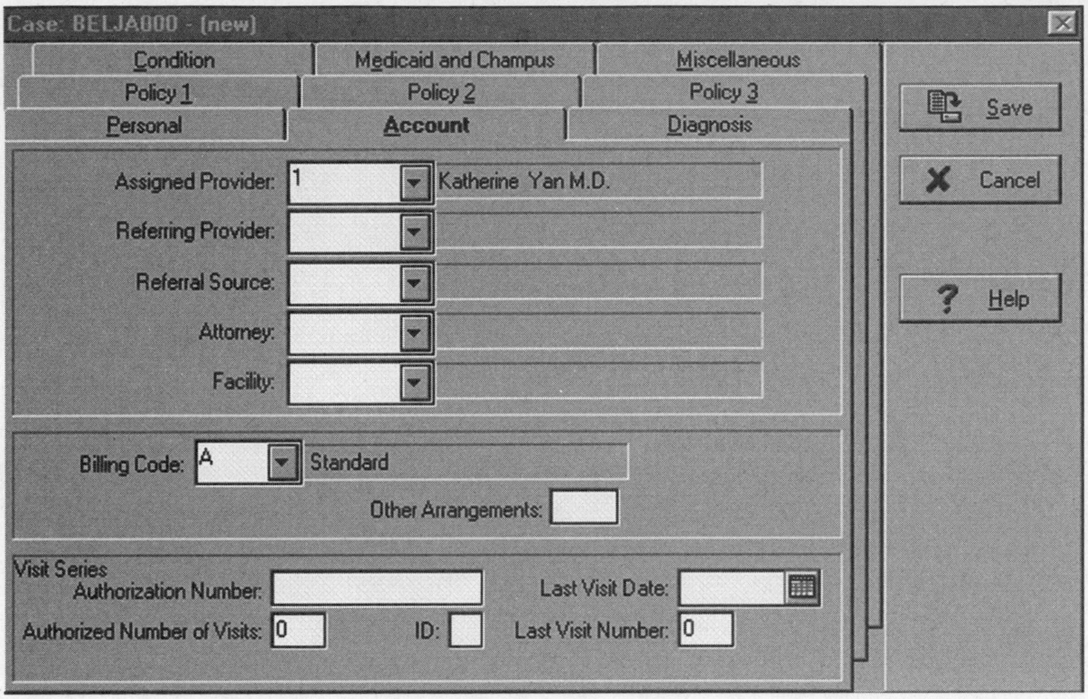

Figure 4-4 *Case Window (Account Folder)*

The *Diagnosis* folder also provides space for you to indicate any allergies or EMC notes. The **EMC** (or Electronic Media Claims) notes field lets you enter pertinent information concerning electronic claims issues.

Policy 1, Policy 2, and Policy 3 Although most patients have only one insurance policy, some patients have several different policies with varying coverage. For example, a retired person may be covered by Medicare as her primary insurance. However, she may also have a supplemental policy to cover those expenses not reimbursed by Medicare.

Using the *Policy* folders, you can enter information for up to three different insurance policies. Most of the fields in the three folders are identical except that Policy 1 asks for a co-payment amount and a capitated plan indicator. (See Figure 4-5, page 72.) For the second policy, you need to indicate whether or not there is any crossover between two of the policies. For example, a primary carrier (usually Medicare) will automatically forward any unpaid portion of a claim to the secondary carrier.

Some insurance policies have patients pay a co-payment amount for each office visit or other service performed. The patient's insurance company pays the remainder of the bill directly to the provider. The **co-payment** is a standard fee ($5.00, $10.00, or $20.00) paid to the provider by a patient for medical services rendered. A **capitated plan** is a type of insurance that pays providers a fixed amount for each patient regardless of the actual services rendered.

Figure 4-5 *Case Window (Policy 1 Folder)*

When you complete a patient's policy information, you must identify the insured party and the relationship to the patient. For a single person with his/her own policy, the insured person is the patient. And, the relationship to the insured would be indicated as "self." Suppose that a child is a patient. In this instance, you would most likely identify a parent as the insured party and the relationship would be noted as "child." Other important information needed to complete a *Policy* folder includes: insurance carrier, assignment acceptance, policy number, group number, policy dates, and insurance coverage percent.

Condition   You can store information related to a patient's illness or injury in the *Condition* folder. In this folder you can include data such as first consultation date, last X-ray date, and Workers' Compensation information.

Medicaid and Champus   Use the *Medicaid and Champus* folder to record related information such as submission numbers, references, and effective dates. For patients covered by Medicaid, you can also indicate if additional coverage is provided by **EPSDT** (a well-baby program) or Family Planning. If a patient is covered by Champus, you can list the branch of service (e.g., Air Force, Army, Marines, etc.) and the sponsor status (e.g., 100% disabled, civilian, active duty, etc.).

Miscellaneous   The *Miscellaneous* folder lets you indicate outside lab work and charges. There are other fields to record extra information about a patient. As with other fields in the case record, these fields are optional.

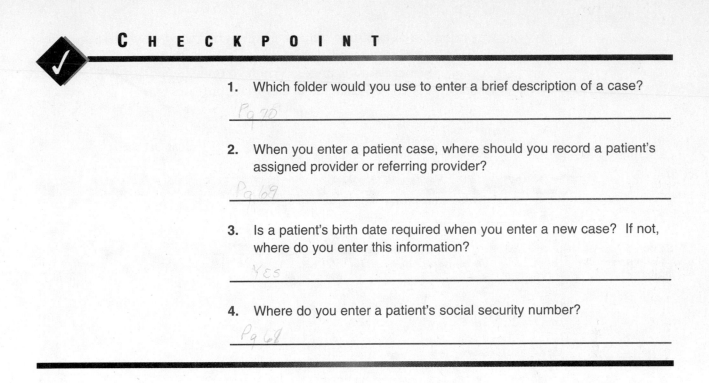

1. Which folder would you use to enter a brief description of a case?

    _Pg 70_

2. When you enter a patient case, where should you record a patient's assigned provider or referring provider?

    _Pg 69_

3. Is a patient's birth date required when you enter a new case? If not, where do you enter this information?

    Yes

4. Where do you enter a patient's social security number?

    _Pg 68_

ENTERING PATIENT AND CASE DATA

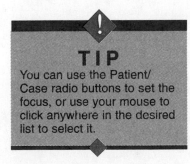

TIP
You can use the Patient/Case radio buttons to set the focus, or use your mouse to click anywhere in the desired list to select it.

MediSoft makes it easy to enter a new patient record, edit existing data, or delete a patient record. And, once you add a new patient to the patient file, filling in the case information is also a straightforward process.

To enter the information you read about in this chapter, use the *Patients/Guarantors and Cases* option in the Lists menu. When you choose this option, the *MediSoft* program displays the Patient List window. As shown in Figures 4-6 and 4-7, page 74, the patient list appears on the left side of the window, and the case list appears on the right side of the window. When the patient list is in focus as shown in Figure 4-6, the Edit Patient, New Patient, and Delete Patient buttons appear at the bottom of the window. The radio buttons at the top of the window indicate the current focus.

Just click the **New Patient** button to begin adding a new patient to the data file. If you need to edit or delete a patient record, first select the desired patient and then click the corresponding button. You can select a patient record by searching for it or by scrolling through the list and clicking a patient's chart number.

The case records that appear on the right side of the Patient List window are linked to the selected patient. (See Figure 4-7.) Only those cases entered for the selected patient appear in the list. Remember that you must set the focus to the Case list before the program displays the buttons shown in Figure 4-7.

To work with patient case records, first locate and select a patient record. Then, click the **New Case** button to add a new case for that patient. To save time, you can highlight an existing case and click the **Copy Case** button to make a copy of a case record. Then, just make the necessary changes. When you need to edit or delete a case, select it and then click the appropriate button.

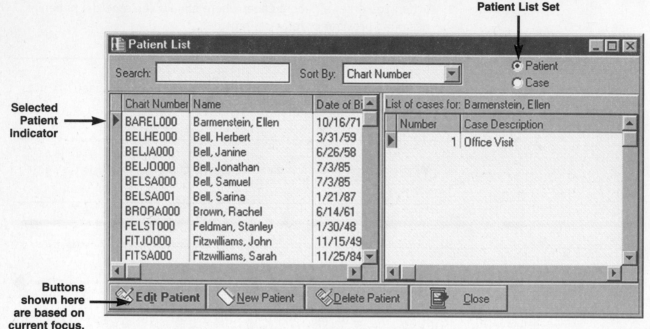

Figure 4-6 *Patient List Window with Patient Selected*

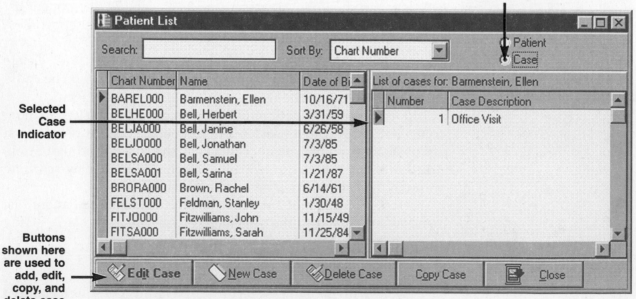

Figure 4-7 *Patient List Window with Case Selected*

CHECKPOINT

5. Which application menu option should you choose to add a new patient record?

P/G CASES   L PG 73

6. Which button can you choose to duplicate an existing case?

COPY CASE   PG 74

7. Does the *MediSoft* program automatically assign a case number or can you set it manually?

YES

8. Which button in the Patient List window lets you change a patient's address?

EDIT Pat

PRACTICE EXERCISE 4-1

Adding a New Patient and Case Record (Juan Lomos)

Follow the steps provided below and on pages 76-77 to add a new patient and case record.

1. Start the *MediSoft* software. Refer to the instructions on page 33 if you need assistance.

2. Set the program date to **September 4, 1998**.

3. Select the *Patients/Guarantors and Cases* option from the Lists menu. Or, use the toolbar to select this option (Patient List button). When you choose this option, the Patient List window appears.

4. Juan Lomos, a new patient, completed the Patient Information form (Source Document 1, page 159). Review the information provided on the form.

5. To add a new patient, click the **New Patient** button provided in the Patient List window.

6. Using the information on Source Document 1, enter the patient's name, address, phone number, birth date, gender, and social security number in the *Name, Address* folder. **Note:** You don't need to enter a chart number; the *MediSoft* program will automatically assign this number.

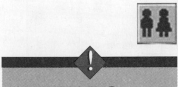

TIPS

Make sure the patient list is selected. Check the radio buttons at the top of the window.

◆

When you enter the phone number, don't enter the parentheses or the hyphen. Just enter **6142210202**. The software will automatically format the phone number. Enter the birth date as **072141**. For the social security number, however, you must enter the hyphens.

7. Switch to the *Other Information* folder.

8. Verify that the *Type* field is set to Patient and enter the assigned provider from the source document.

9. Click on the **Employer** combo box. As you can see, Juan's employer, Stephenson Wire Works, is not listed. You need to add his employer to the Address list before you can continue.

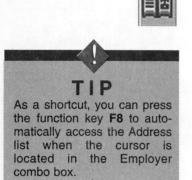

10. Choose the *Addresses* option from the Lists menu, and then click the **New** button.

11. Enter the address information for Stephenson Wire Works in the Address window. Use **15** for the employer code. Then, click the **Save** button in the Address window to save this new record. Close the Address List window, if necessary.

TIP

As a shortcut, you can press the function key **F8** to automatically access the Address list when the cursor is located in the Employer combo box.

12. Now you can complete the employer information (code, status, and work phone).

13. Review the information you entered in the *Name, Address* and *Other Information* folders. (See Figure 4-8 below.) If you notice a mistake, correct the error.

14. Click the **Save** button to save the new patient information. The program will assign the chart number when it saves the record.

Figure 4-8 *New Patient/Guarantor Window (Juan Lomos)*

15. Locate the new record you just added. It should be the selected patient in the Patient List window. If Juan Lomos is not selected, click on his record to select it.

16. Switch the focus so that you can enter the case information for Juan Lomos. Click on the **Case** radio button or click on the right side of the Patient List window.

17. Click the **New Case** button.

18. In the *Personal* folder, enter the following information from Source Document 1: case description, guarantor, marital status, and student status.

    Use the information written on the source document in the *Reason for Visit* field to complete the *Description* field in the data entry window. As shown on Juan's Patient Information form, he is the insured person. Therefore, this also makes him the guarantor. The employment information should already be included in the folder.

19. Switch to the *Account* folder. Several of the fields should already contain data that the *MediSoft* program gathers from other data files. Verify the assigned provider and billing code information.

20. Select the *Policy 1* folder.

21. Enter Juan's chart number to indicate that he is the insured party and set the *Relationship to Insured* field to **Self**.

22. Record Juan's policy information: Insurance (**Blue Cross/Blue Shield**), policy number (**716830061**), group number (**126**), and insurance coverage percent (**80**).

23. Switch to the *Condition* folder.

24. Since Juan's visit was due to an automobile accident, you need to enter this information in the *Condition* folder. Enter the accident date (**8/9/98**) in the *Injury/Illness/LMP Date* field. Set the *Accident, Related To* field to **Auto** and enter **OH** in the *Accident, State* field. **Note:** LMP is an acronym for last menstrual period.

25. Use the additional information prepared by Dr. Yan (Source Document 2, page 161) to complete the *Total Disability, Partial Disability*, and *Hospitalization* date fields in the *Condition* folder.

26. Review the information you entered in each of the folders. (See Figure 4-9 at the top of the next page for the *Personal folder*.) Make any needed corrections.

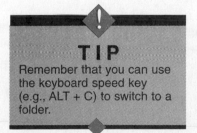

TIP

Remember that you can use the keyboard speed key (e.g., ALT + C) to switch to a folder.

Case: Auto accident--back injury

Condition	Medicaid and Champus	Miscellaneous
Policy 1	Policy 2	Policy 3
Personal	Account	Diagnosis

Case Number: [   ]   ☐ Case Closed

Description: [Auto accident--back injury]

Guarantor: [LOMJU000 ▼] Lomos, Juan

☑ Print Patient Statement

Marital Status: [Married ▼]   Student Status: [Non-student ▼]

Employment

Employer: [15 ▼] Stephenson Wire Works

Status: [Full time ▼]

Retirement Date: [🗓]   Work Phone: [(614)525-0215]

Location: [   ]   Extension: [   ]

Buttons: 🖫 Save | ✕ Cancel | ? Help

Figure 4-9 *New Case/Personal Folder (Juan Lomos)*

27. Save the case information. When you click the **Save** button, the *MediSoft* program will automatically assign a case number.

28. Verify that a case record for Juan Lomos appears in the Patient List window.

PRACTICE EXERCISE 4-2

Adding a New Patient (Cedera Lomos)
Follow the steps provided here to add a new patient and case record for Juan Lomos' wife, Cedera. Review the information she recorded on the Patient Information form (Source Document 3, page 163.)

TIP
Remember that you have to set the focus to "Patient" before you can choose to add a new patient.

1. Click the **New Patient** button to begin entering the new patient information for Cedera Lomos.

2. From the Patient Information form that Cedera completed (Source Document 3), enter the information in the *Name*, *Address* and *Other Information* folders.

3. Review the information you entered, correct any errors, and then save the new patient record.

4. Change the focus to "Case" and then click the **New Case** button to add a new case for Cedera Lomos.

5. Complete the case folders, review your work, and then save the information.

◆ Enter the information for the *Personal* folder. Since Cedera indicated that her husband's insurance is the primary policy, make sure that you select Juan Lomos as the guarantor.

◆ Verify the information in the *Account* folder.

◆ Enter the primary insurance information in the *Policy 1* folder. Be sure to enter **Juan Lomos** as the insured party and enter **Spouse** in the *Relationship to Insured* field. Select **Blue Cross/Blue Shield** for the insurance and enter the other pertinent data.

◆ Record the secondary insurance information in the *Policy 2* folder. In this instance, Cedera is the insured party and the relationship is "self." Enter the insurance company (**Physician Alliance of Ohio**), policy number (**621382**), group number (**A435**), and the coverage percent (**90**).

◆ Make a note of Cedera's allergy to penicillin. Enter this information in the *Diagnosis* folder.

◆ Save the case data.

PRACTICE EXERCISE 4-3

Adding a New Patient (Lisa Lomos)
Follow the steps listed on page 78 and above to add a new patient and case record for Juan and Cedera Lomos' daughter, Lisa. Review the information recorded on her Patient Information form (Source Document 4, page 165.)

1. Record the patient information for Lisa Lomos.

2. Review your work and then save the patient data.

3. Complete the case information that is shown on Lisa's Patient Information form.

4. Check the information you entered and then save the new case record.

PRACTICE EXERCISE 4-4

Adding a New Patient (Angela Wong)
Follow the steps you learned in the previous practice exercises to add a new patient record and case for Angela Wong. Review the information she recorded on the Patient Information form (Source Document 5, page 167.)

IMPORTANT: Angela is a full-time student who is covered by her father's insurance. Her father, Peter Wong, is the guarantor and the insured party. Since her father is not a patient at the Family Care Center, you will have to enter him as a guarantor before you can complete the case information for Angela. The steps to add a guarantor are the same as those for adding a new patient. The only exception is that you don't have to enter some of the information such as birth date, social security number, and employment information. For the *Type* field in the *Other Information* folder, choose "Guarantor" instead of "Patient" for Peter Wong.

PRACTICE EXERCISE 4-5

Editing a Patient Record (John Fitzwilliams)

An existing patient, John Fitzwilliams, changed jobs. Previously, he was self-employed. Review the information on Source Document 6 (page 169). Then, follow these steps to edit Mr. Fitzwilliams' patient record.

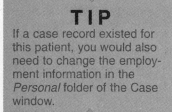

1. Select the *Patients/Guarantors and Cases* option from the Lists menu if the Patient List window is not displayed. Or, use the toolbar to select this option.

2. Make sure the patient list (left side of the window) is in focus.

3. Use the Search feature or scroll through the patient list to select John Fitzwilliams' record.

4. Click the **Edit Patient** button to edit the patient's data.

5. Switch to the *Other Information* folder.

6. Change the employment information as indicated on Source Document 6.

7. Save the changes you made.

> **TIP**
> If a case record existed for this patient, you would also need to change the employment information in the *Personal* folder of the Case window.

PRACTICE EXERCISE 4-6

Updating Case Information (Herbert Mitchell)

Follow the steps presented below to update the case information for Herbert Mitchell. (See Source Document 7, page 171.)

1. Select the *Patients/Guarantors and Cases* option from the Lists menu if the Patient List window is not displayed.

2. Make sure the patient list (left side of the window) is in focus.

3. Use the Search feature or scroll through the patient list to select Mr. Mitchell's record.

4. Once you locate and select his record, select the "Shortness of Breath" case by clicking on it.

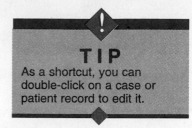

TIP

As a shortcut, you can double-click on a case or patient record to edit it.

5. Click the **Edit Case** button so that you can update the case information.

6. Choose the *Condition* folder and then enter the hospitalization dates shown on Source Document 7.

7. Enter the Medicare authorization number in the *Account* folder.

8. Record the outside lab work in the *Miscellaneous* folder. Be sure to enable the check box and enter the amount.

9. Save the changes you made.

10. Close the Patient List window.

PRACTICE EXERCISE 4-7

Exiting the Program and Making a Backup Disk

Practice quitting the software and making a backup disk by following these steps:

1. Choose *Exit* from the File menu or use the toolbar to select this option.

2. Click the **Exit Program** button in the Backup Reminder window. Do **NOT** choose the backup option.

3. Make a backup copy of your working disk using the *Windows* operating system utilities, not the *MediSoft* option. Follow the instructions on pages 5-6 of the Introduction if you need help making a backup copy using *Windows 3.1* or *Windows 95*.

4. Store your disks in a safe place.

CHAPTER REVIEW

Chapter 4

DEFINE THE TERMS

Write a definition for each term: (Obj. 4-1)

1. Established patient

   _Pg 66_
   _____
   _____
   _____
   _____

2. Billing code

   _Pg 65_
   _____
   _____
   _____
   _____

3. EPSDT

   _Pg 66_
   _____
   _____
   _____
   _____

4. Co-payment

   _Pg 65_
   _____
   _____
   _____
   _____

Chapter 4 ◆ *Entering Patient and Case Information*

CHECK YOUR UNDERSTANDING

5. Which folders in the Case window do you use to enter the insurance information? *(Obj. 4-4)*

_Pg 77_ _____

_____

_____

6. Where do you indicate whether an individual is a patient or a guarantor? Describe a situation where a person would need to be entered into the system as a guarantor, but not as a patient. Can a patient also be a guarantor? Explain. *(Obj. 4-2)*

_Pg 80_ _____

_____

_____

_____

_____

_____

_____

7. What information is recorded in the *Personal* folder of a case record? *(Obj. 4-4)*

_Pg 70_ _____

_____

_____

_____

8. Where would you record a patient's allergy to a prescription drug such as penicillin? *(Obj. 4-4)*

_Pg 70_ _____

_____

_____

_____

9. A patient has Blue Cross/Blue Shield insurance coverage through her employer. She is also covered under her husband's Prudential policy for expenses that Blue Cross/Blue Shield does not cover. How do you enter information on her insurance? *(Obj. 4-5)*

pg 71

_____

_____

_____

_____

 THINK IT THROUGH

10. When might you delete a patient from a medical practice's database? What factors would keep you from deleting a patient account? *(Obj. 4-7)*

_____

_____

_____

_____

_____

_____

_____

_____

Chapter 4 ◆ *Entering Patient and Case Information*

Chapter 5

PROCESSING TRANSACTIONS

WHAT YOU NEED TO KNOW

To complete this chapter, you need to know how to:

- ◆ Use the computer keyboard to enter information in *Medi-Soft*.

- ◆ Navigate the *MediSoft* software.

- ◆ Search for information in a *MediSoft* database.

- ◆ Enter patient and case information.

WHAT YOU WILL LEARN

When you finish this chapter, you will be able to:

1. Define the terms introduced in this chapter.

2. Explain the information contained on a patient's superbill and how it is used to record a transaction.

3. Enter procedure charge transactions.

4. Record payments received from patients and insurance carriers.

5. Print a walkout receipt.

6. Describe how to enter an adjustment.

KEY TERMS

Adjustment   An amount, positive or negative, entered to correct a patient's account balance.

Charge   Amount (or cost) of a procedure performed by a provider.

Default	An entry automatically displayed in an input field.
Diagnosis	A doctor's opinion about a patient's medical condition based on an examination.
EMC Assignment	EMC (Electronic Media Claims) method to process claims electronically.
Inpatient	Reference to a patient treated in a hospital for one or more days.
Outpatient	Reference to a patient who is treated at a hospital, but who does not stay overnight.
Payment	Cash or check sent by a patient or insurance carrier for services rendered.
Transaction	A charge to a patient's account for services rendered, a payment by a patient or insurance carrier, or an adjustment.

HANDLING TRANSACTIONS ➤

During a typical day, many patients visit a medical practice such as the Family Care Center. And, for each patient, the assigned provider will perform specific procedures related to that patient's condition. The physician records on each patient's superbill the procedures performed. In turn, the billing assistant uses the completed superbill as a source document to enter the procedure charge(s). A **charge** is the cost that a medical office assigns to a procedure.

A billing assistant must process **payments**—cash or checks received for medical services rendered—on a daily basis. Some patients make payments immediately after a visit, while others send their payments later by mail. Insurance companies also send payments for covered procedures on the behalf of patients.

On occasion, it may be necessary to make an adjustment to a patient's account. An **adjustment** is an amount (positive or negative) entered to correct a patient's account balance. An adjustment might be required, for example, if an insurance company did not pay as much as expected.

As you will learn in this chapter, the *MediSoft* program can be used to process several different kinds of **transactions**—charges, payments, and adjustments. First, you will learn how to record and enter procedure charges. Then, you will learn how to process payments and adjustments.

For every procedure performed, a billing assistant must make sure that the appropriate information is properly recorded in the patient accounting system. Recording the procedure charges properly is an important first step in the billing cycle. Activities such as managing cash flow, collecting payments, processing claims, and generating reports depend on this first step.

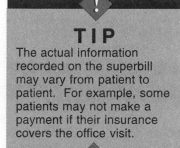

TIP

The actual information recorded on the superbill may vary from patient to patient. For example, some patients may not make a payment if their insurance covers the office visit.

Reviewing a Completed Superbill

As you learned in a previous chapter, the completed superbill is the primary source of information that a billing assistant needs to record procedure charges. As shown in Figure 5-1, page 90, this completed superbill includes the following: provider's name, patient's name and chart number, date the services were performed, procedures performed, payments received, diagnosis, today's charges, remarks, and the next scheduled appointment.

After a physician completes a patient examination, he or she will place a check mark next to those procedures performed. As you may recall, the superbill includes only the most common procedures provided by a medical office. If the physician performs a procedure not listed on the superbill, he or she writes the procedure in the "Other Procedures" area on the form. In these instances, you will have to search for and enter the procedure code when processing a charge.

Many insurance carriers will not pay for treatment without a diagnosis. The **diagnosis** is the doctor's opinion of a patient's condition. Therefore, the doctor must record this information on the superbill so that it can be included as part of the procedure charge. When you enter the diagnosis, you will use the ICD-9 codes as a standard way to record this information.

Entering a Procedure Charge

After you review a patient's superbill, you are ready to enter the transaction to record the procedure charge. You will process all transactions (charges, payments, and adjustments) using the *Enter Transactions* option in the Activities menu. Selecting this option displays the Transaction Entry window. As you can see in Figure 5-2, page 91, transactions are case-based. That is, every transaction, including charges, must be assigned to a patient and a specific case. You cannot enter or edit a transaction until you enter a chart number and a case number.

When you enter procedure charges, you must enter a separate transaction for each charge rather than combining all procedures

Family Care Center
285 Stephenson Boulevard
Stephenson, OH 60089
(614) 555-0100

Provider: Dr. Katherine Yan   **ID #:** 84021   **S.S. #:** 810-99-1110

Patient: *Burke, Jared*   **Chart #:** *BURJA000*   **Document:**

Address: **Phone:**   **Date:** *8/27/98*

CODE	DESCRIPTION	X
New Patient		
99201	OF—New Patient Focused	
99202	OF—New Patient Expanded	
99203	OF—New Patient, Complete Physical	
Established Patient		
99213	OF—Established Patient Expanded	
99214	OF—Established Patient Routine Exam	✓
99215	OF—Established Patient Complex	
99211	OF—Established Patient Minimal	
99212	OF—Established Patient Focused	
Procedures		
85007	Manual WBC	
85651	Erythrocyte Sed Rate—ESR	
86403	Strep Test, Rapid	
86585	Tine Test	
87072	Strep Culture	
87086	Urine Culture	
93000	Electroencephalogram—EEG	✓
93015	Treadmill Stress Test	
90782	Injection	
Other Procedures		
	Glucose—quantitative	✓

Payments: *Received $65, Check #2312*

Diagnosis/ICD-9: *Hyperglycemia*

Remarks: **Today's Charges:** $ *170.00*

Next Appointment: *September 12, 1998*   **Amount Paid:** $ *65.00*

Figure 5-1 *Completed Superbill*

into one single transaction. This step is required since you must provide detailed information about each charge including a description and an amount.

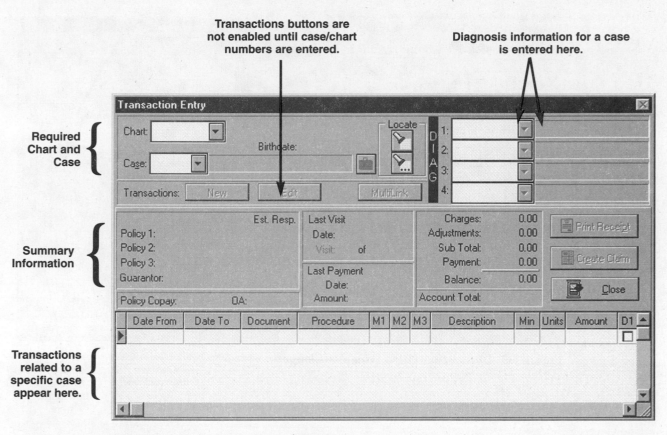

Figure 5-2 *Transaction Entry Window*

Once you enter a chart number and a case number, you can choose to enter a new transaction by clicking the **New** button. When you click this button, the *MediSoft* program displays three folders—*Charge, Payment,* and *Adjustment*. The *Charge* folder appears first as shown in Figure 5-3, page 92. As you can see, the program provides default information in several of the fields. A **default** is an entry that automatically appears in a field and will be accepted unless you change the information.

To record a procedure charge, you need to enter the transaction date and a document number. By default the program enters the current date and also supplies a document number. The program also records default information in the *Provider* field. Usually, you do not have to change these fields.

Next, you must identify the procedure by using its corresponding code. These codes appear on the superbill for the most common procedures. In some instances, you may have to search for the code based on the procedure information written on the superbill. When you enter a procedure code, the *MediSoft* program automatically fills

Records transaction and closes entry area.

Saves transaction and then displays a new entry area.

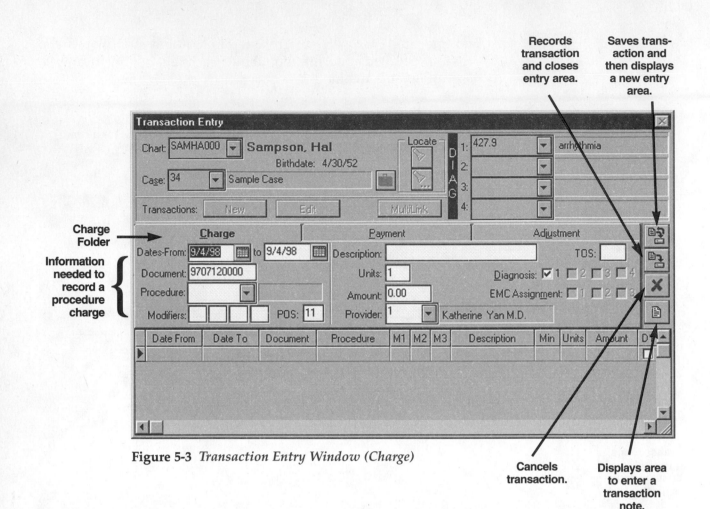

Charge Folder

Information needed to record a procedure charge

Figure 5-3 *Transaction Entry Window (Charge)*

Cancels transaction.

Displays area to enter a transaction note.

in the *Amount*, *POS* (place of service), and *TOS* (type of service) fields based on the information stored in the Procedure data file. Usually, you do not have to change this information. After you record a procedure code, you can enter additional information in the *Modifiers* fields to further define a procedure.

As part of the charge transaction data, you need to identify the place (or location) where a procedure took place. Although most procedures take place in the office, some patients may receive inpatient or outpatient care. **Inpatient** refers to care provided when patients must stay overnight at a hospital. **Outpatient**, on the other hand, refers to medical care provided at a hospital, but the patient does not stay overnight. Use the *POS* (place of service) field to enter a code that identifies the location for the procedure.

To complete the information needed to record a charge, you must enter a description, units (or quantity), diagnosis, and EMC assignment. For the description, you can enter an explanation of the procedure or use the diagnosis. Leave the *Units* field set to 1 unless stated otherwise. The *Diagnosis* check boxes correspond to the diagnosis information shown in the upper portion of the Transaction Entry window. This field lets you link a procedure to a particular diagnosis. The **EMC Assignment** (or Electronic

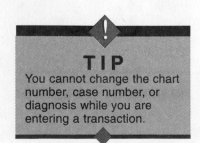

TIP
You cannot change the chart number, case number, or diagnosis while you are entering a transaction.

Media Claims) check boxes are used when a medical office processes its claims electronically. These options are not used in this tutorial.

Once you record the required information, the last step is to save the information you entered. Then, if there is another procedure charge, you repeat the same steps. After you record the last procedure, you can review the transaction data provided in the summary area. The summary area includes the procedure charge total, adjustments, payments, and account total. Information is also included regarding the estimated amount to be paid by the patient's insurance company.

Printing a Walkout Receipt and Creating a Claim

After you complete a transaction, the *MediSoft* program makes it easy to print a receipt for a customer and generate an insurance claim. Just click the **Print Receipt** button to print a detailed receipt similar to the receipt shown in Figure 5-4, p. 94. The patient information (i.e., name, diagnosis, charges, and amounts) pertaining to the case appears on the printout.

Generating the information needed to produce an insurance claim form is also a simple process. You can click the **Create Claim** button in the Transaction Entry window to create a claim immediately, or you can create claims later as you will learn in Chapter 7. When you create a claim, the *MediSoft* program gathers the necessary information from the data you entered and stores it so that you can print an insurance form such as the HCFA-1500 or send the information electronically.

✓ C H E C K P O I N T

1. Which application menu option do you use to enter a procedure charge?

   Pg 89

2. What document is the primary source of information that is used to record a procedure charge transaction?

   Pg 11 & 91

3. What two pieces of information must be entered before you can enter a procedure charge?

   Pg 89

Family Care Center
285 Stephenson Boulevard
Stephenson, OH 60089
(614) 555-0100

Patient: Cedera Lomos
12 Briar Lane
Stephenson, OH 60089

Diagnosis: 1. 473.9   sinusitis–chronic
2.
3.
4.

Account Number: LOMCE000
    Case #: 25

Instructions: Complete the patient information portion of your own insurance claim form. Attach this bill, signed and dated, and all other bills pertaining to the claim. If you have a deductible policy, hold your claim forms until you have met your deductible. Mail directly to your insurance carrier.

Date	Description	Procedure	Modify	DX	Units	Charge
9/4/98	OF–New patient, mod. complex	99204		1	1	100.00

Provider information

Provider Name: Katherine Yan, M.D.
License: 84021
Blue Cross/Shield PIN: 60-3872-8
Social Security #: 810-99-1110

Total Charges: 100.00
Total Credits: 0.00
Total Due This Visit: 100.00
Total Balance Due: 100.00

Assign and Release: I hereby authorize payment of medical benefits to this physician for the services described above. I also authorize the release of any information necessary to process this claim.

Patient Signature: _____ **Date:** _____

Figure 5-4 *Walkout Receipt*

PRACTICE EXERCISE 5-1

Entering a Patient Charge Transaction (Cedera Lomos)

The superbill for Cedera Lomos is shown in Source Document 8 (page 173). Record the procedure charge and the diagnosis by following these steps:

1. Start the *MediSoft* program.

2. Set the program date to **September 4, 1998**.

3. Select the *Enter Transactions* option from the Activities menu. Or, use the toolbar to select this option. When you choose this option, the Transaction Entry window appears.

4. Review the information shown on the superbill in Source Document 8. As you can see, there is one procedure charge (OF—New Patient, Mod. Complex) and a diagnosis (sinusitis—chronic) written on the superbill.

5. In the Transaction Entry window, select Cedera's chart number and then choose the case number for this visit.

6. Use the mouse to click in the first diagnosis field in the upper right corner of the Transaction Entry window. Enter the diagnosis code for sinusitis—chronic. Scroll through the list to find the diagnosis.

7. Click the **New** button to begin entering the procedure charge for Cedera Lomos.

8. Accept the default information shown in the date fields. The dates should be September 4, 1998 **(9/4/98).**

9. Accept the default document number.

10. Enter the procedure code **(99204)** for New Patient, Mod. Complex in the *Procedure* field. Notice that the charge amount ($100.00) is automatically filled in when you enter the procedure code and accept it by moving out of the field.

11. Leave the *Modifiers* fields empty.

12. Accept the information in the *POS* (place of service) field. The code should be set to **11** since this is the default code.

13. Enter **Office visit** in the *Description* field.

14. Accept **1** for the units.

15. Verify that the *Amount* field is set to $100.00. If not, first check that you entered the procedure code correctly. If it is correct, accept the amount.

16. Accept the provider information. This field should already include the provider code for Dr. Yan.

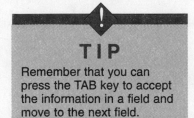

TIP

Remember that you can press the TAB key to accept the information in a field and move to the next field.

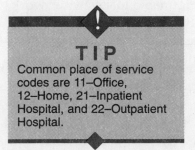

TIP

Common place of service codes are 11–Office, 12–Home, 21–Inpatient Hospital, and 22–Outpatient Hospital.

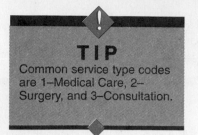

TIP

Common service type codes are 1–Medical Care, 2–Surgery, and 3–Consultation.

17. Accept the information in the *TOS* (type of service) field. Code 1 (medical care) is the default code for this field.

18. For each charge, you need to identify a corresponding diagnosis. Since there was only one diagnosis, the program automatically selects it. Verify that the first Diagnosis check box is selected.

19. Since Family Care Center does not process claims electronically, the *EMC* (Electronic Media Claims) *Assignment* fields should not be selected.

20. Compare the information you entered for the charge to the data shown in Figure 5-5. Correct any errors, if necessary.

Saves and closes transaction

Transaction Entry

Chart: LOMCE000 ▼ **Lomos, Cedera**   Locate   1: 473.9 ▼ sinusitis - chronic
Birthdate: 5/21/46   2:
Case: 25 ▼ Persistent cough   3:
Transactions: New   Edit   MultiLink   4:

Charge Folder →

| **Charge** | Payment | Adjustment |

Dates-From: 9/4/98 to 9/4/98   Description: Office visit   TOS: 1
Document: 9809040000   Units: 1   Diagnosis: ☑1 ☐2 ☐3 ☐4
Procedure: 99204 ▼ OF--New   Amount: 100.00   EMC Assignment: ☐1 ☐2 ☐3
Modifiers: POS: 11   Provider: 1 ▼ Katherine Yan M.D.

Date From	Date To	Document	Procedure	M1	M2	M3	Description	Min	Units	Amount	D1
9/4/98	9/4/98	9809040000	99204				Office visit		1	100.00	☒

Figure 5-5 *Transaction Entry (Charge Transaction)*

21. Click the **Save** button identified in Figure 5-5 to save your work and close the entry area. The other Save button above saves the transaction and automatically opens another transaction entry window. Since there is only one transaction for this patient, you don't need to use this button.

22. When you save a transaction, the *MediSoft* program updates the information (policy, charges, payments, last visit, and account total) shown in the Transaction Entry screen. (See Figure 5-6.)

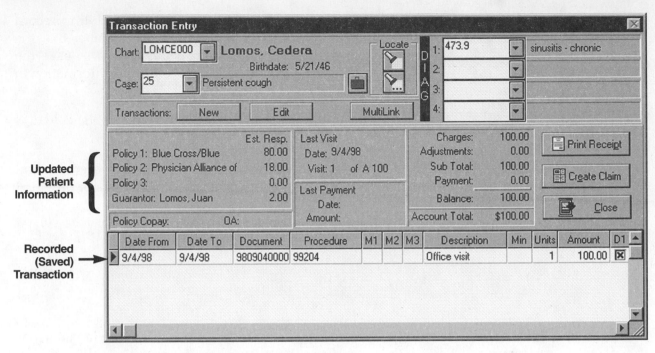

Figure 5-6 *Transaction Entry (Completed)*

23. Click the **Print Receipt** button and choose to print a walkout receipt for Cedera Lomos.

24. Close the Transaction Entry window if you are finished, or leave it open to enter the next transaction described in Practice Exercise 5-2.

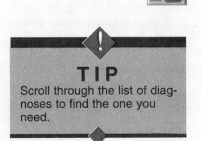

PRACTICE EXERCISE 5-2

Entering a Patient Charge Transaction (Lisa Lomos)

Record the procedure charge information for Lisa Lomos. The superbill completed by Dr. Yan is shown in Source Document 9 (page 175). As you can see, there are two procedures marked on this superbill and two diagnoses. The "normal state" diagnosis is linked to the "complete physical" procedure. The "immunization" diagnosis is a result of the "MMR" (measles, mumps, and rubella) procedure.

1. Select the *Enter Transactions* option from the Activities menu if the Transaction Entry window is not on your screen. Or, use the toolbar to select this option.

2. Enter the chart number for Lisa Lomos and then select the case for her well-child checkup.

TIP
Scroll through the list of diagnoses to find the one you need.

3. Enter both of the diagnoses in the spaces provided. Enter the "normal state" diagnosis first.

4. Click the **New** button to record a new charge transaction.

Chapter 5 ◆ *Processing Transactions*

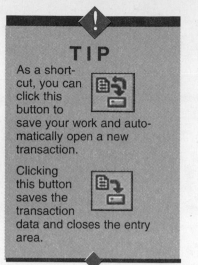
5. Enter the transaction information from the superbill to record the complete physical procedure charge. Remember that the "normal state" diagnosis is linked to this charge. Leave the default fields as they are unless you have specific information to change them.

6. Save the charge transaction information. Then, choose to add another new transaction.

7. Enter and save the information for the MMR procedure. You will have to look up the procedure since a code is not provided on the superbill.

8. Check your work. The account total should be $218.00 for Lisa Lomos.

9. Print a walkout receipt.

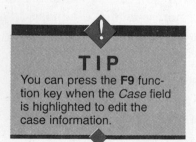

PRACTICE EXERCISE 5-3

Entering a Patient Charge and Adding a New Case (Leila Patterson)
Review the superbill for Leila Patterson shown in Source Document 10 (page 177). Leila is an established patient who made an appointment to have her cholesterol checked. During the office visit, Dr. Yan performed two procedures for this patient, both of which are linked to the one diagnosis. **Note:** Ms. Patterson does not have health insurance.

Follow the steps below to enter a patient charge and create a new case.

1. Enter Leila Patterson's chart number in the Transaction Entry window. When you enter her chart number, a default case code does not appear since there are no case records already entered for Leila.

2. Move to the *Case* field.

3. As a shortcut, press the **F8** function key to begin entering a new case. Another way to enter a new case would be to use the *Patients/Guarantors and Cases* option in the Lists menu, but the shortcut is much faster.

4. Complete the *Description* field in the *Personal* case folder. Enter the diagnosis for the description. Since you don't have any other information at this time and Ms. Patterson does not have insurance coverage, you can complete the new case entry by clicking the **Save** button.

5. To accept the new case number, you must press **TAB** or **ENTER** before you can enter a diagnosis or add a new transaction.

6. Enter the diagnosis for this case in the Transaction Entry window.

7. Enter both procedure charge transactions and save your work. Accept the defaults for the information not provided on the superbill. Ms. Patterson's account total should be $90.00.

8. Print a walkout receipt.

PRACTICE EXERCISE 5-4

Entering a Patient Charge and Adding a New Case (Ellen Barmenstein)

Review the superbill for Ellen Barmenstein shown in Source Document 11 (page 179). Follow these steps to record the transaction for this patient.

1. Enter Ellen Barmenstein's chart number in the Transaction Entry window.

2. A case number appears, but today's visit is for another reason. Create a new case for this office visit. Enter a description in the *Personal* folder. In the *Policy 1* folder, enter Ms. Barmenstein as the insured. She is covered by **Physicians Choice Services** (policy: **13056**, group: **K1047**, percent coverage: **80**).

3. Record the diagnosis and then enter the procedure charge transaction.

4. Save your work.

5. Print a walkout receipt.

6. Close the Transaction Entry window.

PROCESSING PAYMENTS AND ADJUSTMENTS

The next step in the billing process is the processing of payments received from patients and insurance companies. Payment transactions are also entered using the *Enter Transactions* option in the Activities menu. Payments, like charges, are case-based. You must enter a patient's chart number and a case number before you can apply a payment to a patient's account.

To record a payment, you must choose to enter a new transaction and then complete the required fields in the *Payment* folder. (See Figure 5-7, p. 100.) You must enter a transaction date, document number, payment code, description, and amount. You must also indicate who made the payment—a patient or an insurance company.

This button allows you to apply a payment to the charges entered for a case.

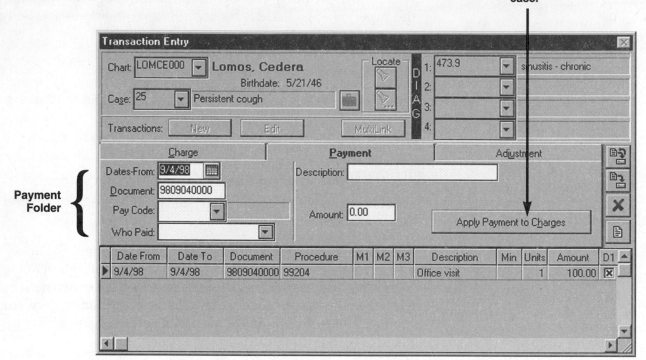

Figure 5-7 *Transaction Entry (Payment)*

One of the final steps in recording a payment is to apply the payment amount to one or more procedure charges. A typical charge could include two procedures ($60.00 and $25.00, for example). If a patient sent a check for $85.00, you must apply $60.00 to the first procedure and the remainder ($25.00) to the other procedure. When an insurance company sends a check for covered services, the health insurance carrier may pay only a partial amount or a percentage of one or more procedure charges. In these cases, you must apply the appropriate amount to each charge.

Occasionally, it may be necessary to make an adjustment to a patient's account. For example, an insurance company may request a refund for a procedure charge that was mistakenly paid. To enter an adjustment, use the *Enter Transactions* option. Enter the patient's chart number and case number. Then, choose to begin a new transaction. Complete the fields in the *Adjustment* folder to record the adjustment. Use a positive or negative amount depending on the nature of the adjustment.

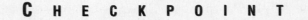

CHECKPOINT

4. Which application menu option do you use to enter a payment?

Pg 99

5. Which option do you use to assign a payment to a particular procedure charge?

Pg 100

6. Which transaction folder would you use to record a check sent by a patient for medical services rendered?

Pg 100

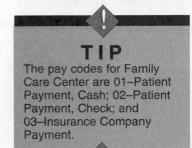

PRACTICE EXERCISE 5-5

Recording a Payment from a Patient for Services Rendered

Elizabeth Jones, a patient, sent Check #1617 for $70.00 for services rendered on August 28, 1998. Follow the steps listed below and on page 102 to record her payment.

1. Select the *Enter Transactions* option from the Activities menu. Or, use the toolbar to select this option.

2. Enter Ms. Jones's chart number.

   Since there is only one case for this patient, the case number automatically appears when you enter the chart number. If there were more than one case, you would have to select the appropriate case to see the corresponding charges.

3. Click the **New** transaction button and then click the *Payment* folder tab to select it.

4. Accept the current date (9/4/98) and the default document number.

5. Enter **02** in the *Pay Code* field for a customer payment made by check.

6. Enter the patient's name in the *Who Paid* field.

7. Record the check number in the *Description* field.

8. Enter the check amount (**70.00**) in the *Amount* field.

> **TIP**
>
> The pay codes for Family Care Center are 01–Patient Payment, Cash; 02–Patient Payment, Check; and 03–Insurance Company Payment.

9. Click the **Apply Payment to Charges** button so that you can apply the $70.00 payment to the appropriate procedure charges.

10. Enter the payment amounts (**60.00** and **10.00**) in the *This Payment* fields shown in the Apply Payment to Charges window. As you can see, there are two procedure charges—one for $60 and the other for $10. The $70 payment covers both charges and must be applied accordingly. (See Figure 5-8. **Note:** The windows have been resized and moved so that you can see the data in both windows at the same time.)

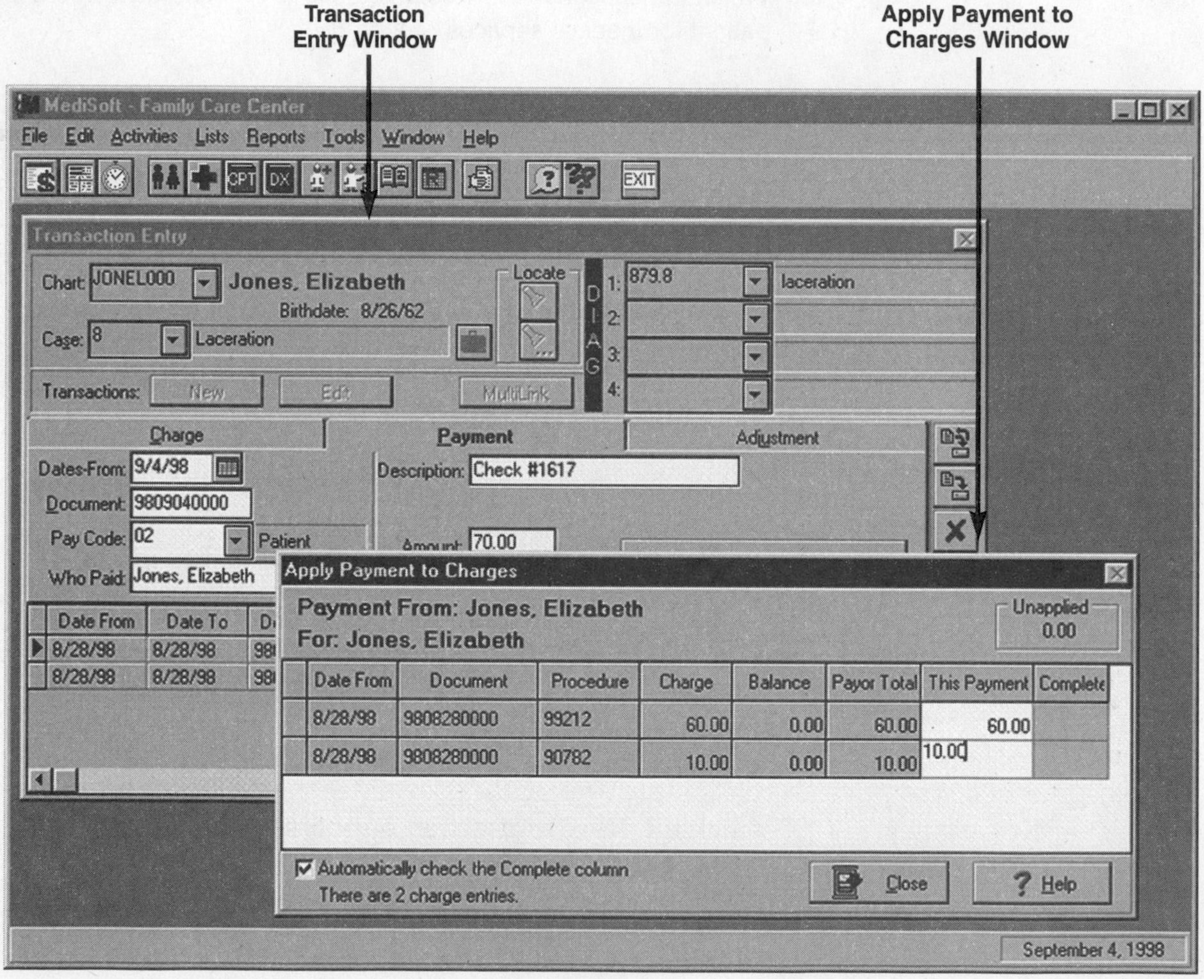

Figure 5-8 *Transaction Entry and Apply Payment to Charges Windows*

11. Click the **Close** button to close the Apply Payment to Charges window after you record the payment. Then save the transaction.

12. Review the information in the updated Transaction Entry window (Figure 5 - 9). If there are any errors, highlight the transaction and then edit the entry.

Notice that the payment is now shown in the lower half of the window. The payment appears as a negative amount (-70.00). Also, you can see that the patient's account total is now $0.00.

**Account
total is $0.00.**

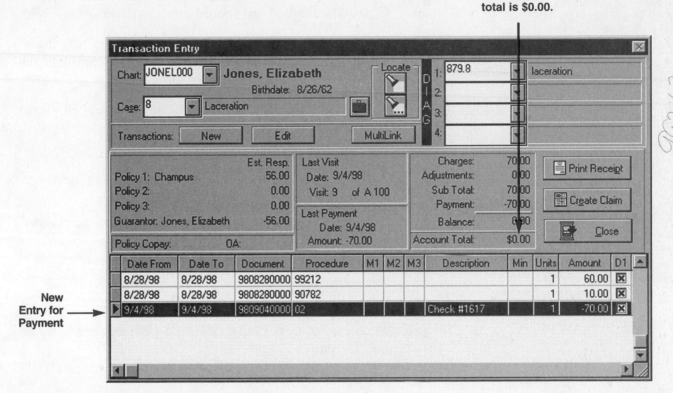

Figure 5-9 *Updated Transaction Entry Window*

**PRACTICE
EXERCISE
5-6**

Recording Payments from Insurance Carriers
Family Care Center received three checks from several of its patients' insurance carriers. Information regarding these payments is listed below and on page 104.

- Hiro Tanaka's insurance carrier (Champus) sent Check #198-9886 in the amount of $162.50 for medical services performed on August 12, 1998. Only a portion of the actual charge was covered. Although you could apply an amount to each procedure charge, apply the entire payment to the first charge. The patient is responsible for the unpaid balance.

- Champus also sent Check #198-9892 in the amount of $500.00 for services rendered for James Smith. The check covers the entire $300.00 charge on July 9 and $200.00 for the August 14 procedure charge.

Chapter 5 ◆ *Processing Transactions*

◆ Physicians Choice Services sent Check #2321332 in the amount of $40.00 for payment of services provided to Ellen Barmenstein on August 28, 1998.

Follow the steps listed below to record the payments:

1. Enter Hiro Tanaka's chart number in the Transaction Entry window. Case **20** (Ankle sprain) should be shown in the *Case* field.

2. When the case information was originally entered, the insurance carrier was not recorded. Before you can complete the payment, you must enter this information.

    ◆ With the *Case* field selected, press the shortcut key **F9** to edit the corresponding case record.

    ◆ Switch to the *Policy 1* folder.

    ◆ Move to the *Insurance 1* field and select **Champus** for the carrier.

    ◆ Click the **Save** button to save the updated case information.

3. Choose to enter a new transaction and then select the *Payment* folder.

4. Accept the date and document number.

5. Enter **03** in the *Pay Code* field to reflect a payment made by an insurance company.

6. Select **Champus** to indicate who paid.

7. Enter the check number for the description.

8. Enter **162.50** for the amount.

9. Click the **Apply Payment to Charges** button.

10. Apply the full payment (**162.50**) to the first procedure charge that was originally billed for $189.50. Then close the window.

11. Save the payment transaction.

12. Verify your work. The patient's account total should now be $137.00.

13. Enter the **$500.00** payment from Champus for James Smith. Refer to the information provided at the beginning of this practice exercise to determine how to apply the payment. Be sure to proof and save your work.

14. Record the **$40.00** payment from Physicians Choice Services for Ellen Barmenstein. **Note:** Two case records are recorded for

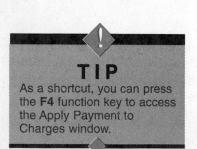

TIP

As a shortcut, you can press the **F4** function key to access the Apply Payment to Charges window.

Ms. Barmenstein. Choose the case that shows the procedure charges on August 28, not the most recent on September 4.

PRACTICE EXERCISE 5-7

Recording a Procedure Charge and Payment from a Patient (Jim Smolowski)

Record the procedure charge and payment from Jim Smolowski as shown on Source Document 12 (page 181). Follow the steps provided below.

1. Enter the chart number for Mr. Smolowski.

2. Move to the *Case* field and press **F8** to enter a new case for this patient.

3. Enter a case description in the *Personal* folder.

4. In the *Policy 1* folder, record the insurance policy information shown below. This information was taken from Mr. Smolowski's Patient Information form that he completed several months ago.

   Insured: Jim Smolowski
   Relationship: self
   Insurance: Physician Alliance of Ohio
   Policy No.: 188383833
   Group No.: 145
   Percent Coverage: 80

5. Save the new case information. Then remember to press **TAB** while in the *Case* field of the Transaction Entry window to accept the case number.

6. Record the diagnosis for the case.

7. Enter and save the procedure charges, which should total $170.00.

8. Enter the payment (**Check #345, $75.00**) paid by the patient as shown on Source Document 12.

   To apply a payment from a patient when there are multiple procedure charges, begin with the first procedure. Apply as much of the payment as possible to the first procedure charge. If there is still an unapplied balance, apply it to the next procedure charge, and so on.

9. Check your work. The account total for Jim Smolowski should be $95.00. Print a walkout receipt for the patient.

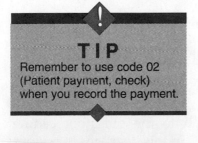

TIP
Remember to use code 02 (Patient payment, check) when you record the payment.

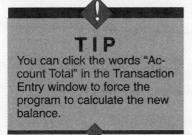

TIP
You can click the words "Account Total" in the Transaction Entry window to force the program to calculate the new balance.

PRACTICE EXERCISE 5-8

Recording a Procedure Charge and Payment from a Patient (Li Yu Wong)

Record the procedure charge and payment from Li Yu Wong as shown on Source Document 13 (page 183). Follow the steps provided here.

1. Enter the chart number for Li Yu Wong.

2. Select Case **23** (Shoulder pain) since the reason for this visit is similar to the previous case.

3. Add a new charge for today's procedure to the existing list of charges for this case.

4. Record the $10.00 cash payment. Apply it to the oldest charge.

5. Verify your work.

6. Print a walkout receipt.

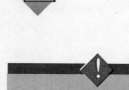

PRACTICE EXERCISE 5-9

Recording a Procedure Charge and Payment from a Patient (Jo Wong)

Record the procedure charge and payment from Jo Wong as shown on Source Document 14 (page 185). Follow the steps provided here.

1. Enter the chart number for Jo Wong.

2. Create a new case since the reason for the visit is different than the previous visit. Enter a description and the insurance information. Mr. Wong is the insured and he is covered by Medicare.

3. Record the diagnosis **(bronchitis, unqualified).**

4. Record the new charges related to this case for today's two procedures.

5. Record the $20.00 payment. Apply it to the previous case. With any payment, you should apply it to the oldest procedure charges unless instructed otherwise. In this instance, a previous case still had an outstanding balance.

6. Verify your work.

7. Make sure that the case to which you applied the payment is selected. Then, print a walkout receipt.

8. Select the new case you just entered and print a walkout receipt for this case, too.

9. Close the Transaction Entry window.

> **TIP**
>
> As a shortcut, you can press the **F8** function key while in the *Case* field to add a new case.

**PRACTICE
EXERCISE
5-10**

Exiting the Program and Making a Backup Disk

Practice quitting the software and making a backup disk by following these steps:

1. Choose *Exit* from the File menu or use the toolbar to select this option.

2. Click the **Exit Program** button in the Backup Reminder window. Do **NOT** choose the backup option.

3. Make a backup copy of your working disk using the *Windows* operating system utilities, not the *MediSoft* option. Follow the instructions on pages 5-6 of the Introduction if you need help making a backup copy using *Windows 3.1* or *Windows 95*.

4. Store your disks in a safe place.

Chapter 5

CHAPTER REVIEW

DEFINE THE TERMS

Write a definition for each term: (Obj. 5-1)

1. Charge

_____

_____

_____

2. Diagnosis

_____

_____

_____

3. Payment

_____

_____

_____

4. Inpatient

_____

_____

_____

5. Adjustment

_____

_____

_____

CHECK YOUR UNDERSTANDING

6. What are the steps required to record a procedure charge? *(Objs. 5-2,3)*

    Pg 99 + 100

7. How do you record a payment from a patient? Why is it necessary to apply the payment to specific charges? *(Obj. 5-4)*

    Pg 100

8. To enter a procedure charge, do you have to identify the patient's chart number and case number? What steps are required if a case has not been set up? *(Obj. 5-3)*

    Pg 98

9. Can you edit the information stored in a patient's case record while working in the Transaction Entry window? Explain. *(Obj. 5-3)*

    Pg 89

10. What information is printed on a walkout receipt? *(Obj. 5-5)*

Pg 93

 THINK IT THROUGH

11. Why does the *MediSoft* program organize transactions based on patient cases? *(Objs. 5-3,4)*

Chapter 6

PRODUCING REPORTS AND PATIENT STATEMENTS

WHAT YOU NEED TO KNOW

To complete this chapter, you need to know how to:

◆ Enter information in *MediSoft*.

◆ Navigate the *MediSoft* software.

◆ Search for information in a *MediSoft* database.

◆ Enter patient and case information.

◆ Record procedure charges and payments.

WHAT YOU WILL LEARN

When you finish this chapter, you will be able to:

1. Define the terms introduced in this chapter.

2. Describe the steps to print a report.

3. Print a Patient Day Sheet and a Procedure Day Sheet.

4. Print a Patient Ledger report.

5. Print a Patient Aging report.

6. Print a Practice Analysis report.

7. Explain the purpose of insurance aging reports.

8. Print Patient Statements.

9. Print various list reports.

10. Describe how to design a custom report.

KEY TERMS

Aging   The classification of accounts receivable by the length of time an account is past due.

Cash flow	Movement of money into a practice from patients and out of a practice to suppliers and staff. Refers to actual cash as opposed to receivables and payables.
Insurance Aging report	Report that shows an aging analysis of insurance accounts.
Patient Aging report	A detailed report that shows an aging analysis of patient accounts.
Patient Statement	Report that shows the services rendered to a patient, total payments, total charges, adjustments, and the balance due.
Payables	Money owed by a practice, but not yet sent to suppliers.
Practice Analysis report	Detailed report that shows the practice's revenue for a period of time.
Receivables	Money owed to a medical practice, but not yet received from patients and insurance companies.

MEDISOFT REPORTS

Reports provide a summary of the data stored in a database such as the one used by *MediSoft* to track patient billing transactions. The reports produced by the *MediSoft* program contain a variety of useful information about a medical practice and its patients.

You as the billing assistant, the office manager, and the providers may have different informational needs for the data provided on the various reports. For example, you might use the Patient Day Sheet to verify a bank deposit since this report shows the cash received during the day. Other reports may help the office manager track the medical practice's **cash flow** or movement of money into and out of the practice.

Information regarding receivables and payables along with aging data is also used to manage the financial aspects of a medical practice. **Receivables**, which represent money owed to a practice by its patients and insurance carriers, must be constantly tracked. Reports that show **aging** data classify receivables by the length of time an account is past due. An office manager could use this data to know which patients or companies have accounts that are past due. **Payables**, or amounts due to suppliers, must be managed, too.

Some of the reports that you can print using the *MediSoft* program are listed below. These reports are described in detail later in this chapter.

◆ Patient Day Sheet

◆ Procedure Day Sheet

- Patient Ledger
- Patient Aging
- Practice Analysis
- Insurance Aging
- Patient Statements
- HCFA-1500
- Lists

DAY SHEETS

Two day sheets were introduced in Chapter 1. These reports summarize activity during a specific period (day, week, or month). Typically, these reports are printed at the end of each day. You can use the reports as a backup for the day's transactions, to verify the cash on hand with the receipts listed on the report, and to analyze the revenue for the day.

The Patient Day Sheet summarizes the procedures, charges, payments, and adjustments by patient. The Procedure Day Sheet provides similar information, but it is organized by procedure codes.

PRACTICE EXERCISE 6-1

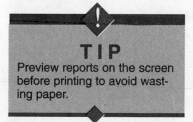

TIP
Preview reports on the screen before printing to avoid wasting paper.

Printing a Patient Day Sheet and a Procedure Day Sheet

1. Start the *MediSoft* program and set the program date to **September 4, 1998.**

2. Pull down the **Reports** menu and choose the *Patient Day Sheet* option.

3. When you see the Print Report Where? dialog box, make sure the *Preview the report on the screen* option is selected.

4. Click the **Start** button.

5. In the *Date From Range* fields, enter **9/4/98** for the beginning and ending dates to print a day sheet for September 4, 1998 only. Then, click the **OK** button.

   After a few moments, the report should appear on your screen as shown in Figure 6-1, page 116. The buttons in the Preview Report window let you zoom the report, move from page to page, print the report, save it to disk, and close the report window.

6. Click the **Zoom to width of page** button so that you can read the report information.

7. Scan the information shown on the report.

8. Click the **Next page** (right arrow) button to view each of the report pages.

9. Click the **Printer** button to print the report.

10. Click the **Close** button to close the Preview Report window.

11. Print a Procedure Day Sheet for September 4, 1998.

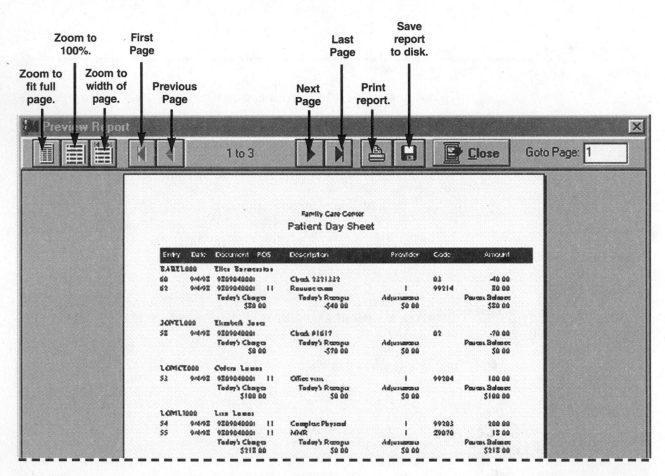

Figure 6-1 *Preview Report Window (Patient Day Sheet)*

ANALYSIS REPORTS

Several reports that can be prepared with the *MediSoft* program are useful in analyzing a medical practice's financial activity. These reports include the following: Patient Ledger, Patient Aging, Insurance Aging, and Practice Analysis. Each report provides a different perspective of the financial data stored in the patient accounting system.

The Patient Ledger report lets you view the account activity for each patient. The ledger includes the procedure charges, payments, and adjustments for all patients or selected patients. It also shows the current balance and any unpaid charges.

Although the Patient Ledger report lets you review patient accounts, this report does not help you determine whether or not patients are paying their bills on time. The **Patient Aging report**, however, shows the "age" for all outstanding patient charges. The report classifies charges using four aging categories—Current (0-30 days), 31-60 days, 61-90 days, and 91 days or older. See the sample Patient Aging report shown in Figure 6-2, page 118. The Patient Aging report is an important tool in collections since you can easily identify patients whose accounts are past due.

The **insurance aging** reports are excellent tools for tracking claims filed with insurance carriers. There are three insurance aging reports: Primary Insurance Aging, Secondary Insurance Aging, and Tertiary Insurance Aging. These reports provide aging information similar to the Patient Aging report. Instead of patients, however, the reports show each insurance carrier and its outstanding balance status.

The **Practice Analysis** report shows the total revenue for each procedure performed during a specific period (e.g., week, month, or year). The summary section of the report includes information such as: total procedure charges, total insurance payments, total patient payments, and net effect on accounts receivable. (See Figure 6-3, page 119.) This report is useful in analyzing which procedures generated the most revenue. Subsequently, the report can be used to perform a profitability analysis and may be helpful to an accountant when preparing financial statements for the medical practice.

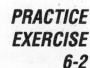

PRACTICE EXERCISE 6-2

Printing Analysis Reports

1. Pull down the **Reports** menu and choose the *Patient Ledger* option.

2. Choose to preview the report on the screen.

3. Click the **Start** button to display the report.

   After you choose to preview the report on the screen, the program displays the Data Selection Questions dialog box. The questions (options) that appear depend on the report you chose. For the Patient Ledger report, for example, you can leave the fields empty to print a report that reflects all of the data stored in the database. However, you could print a Patient Ledger report for only one patient by entering that patient's chart number in the *Chart Number Range* fields. Or,

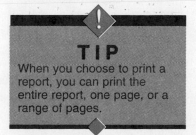

TIP

When you choose to print a report, you can print the entire report, one page, or a range of pages.

Family Care Center
Patient Aging

Chart	Name	–Current– 0-30	–Past– 31-60	–Past– 61-90	–Past–Total 91–>	Balance
BAREL000 (614)274-4242 Last Payment:	**Ellen Barmenstein** -40.00 On: 9/4/98 Patient Aging Totals	 80.00	 0.00	 0.00	 0.00	 $80.00
BELHE000 (614)241-6124 Last Payment:	**Herbert Bell** -60.00 On: 8/28/98 Patient Aging Totals	 150.00	 20.00	 0.00	 0.00	 $170.00
BELSA000 (614)241-6124 Last Payment:	**Samuel Bell** On: Patient Aging Totals	 0.00	 0.00	 0.00	 45.00	 $45.00
BRORA000 (614)721-0044 Last Payment:	**Rachel Brown** On: Patient Aging Totals	 120.00	 0.00	 0.00	 0.00	 $120.00
FELST000 (614)555-9295 Last Payment:	**Stanley Feldman** -75.00 On: 8/23/98 Patient Aging Totals	 0.00	 0.00	 50.00	 0.00	 $50.00
	Practice Aging Total Percent of Aging Total	350.00 75.3%	20.00 4.3%	50.00 10.8%	45.00 9.7%	$465.00 100.0%

Figure 6-2 *Patient Aging Report*

Family Care Center
Practice Analysis

Code	Description	Amount	Quantity	Average	Cost	Net
01	Patient payment, cash	-70.00	4	-17.50		-70.00
02	Patient payment, check	-205.00	3	-68.33		-205.00
03	Insurance Company, payment	-702.50	3	-234.17		-702.50
45380	Colonoscopy—specimen	75.00	1	75.00	0.00	75.00
71010	Chest X ray, frontal	40.00	1	40.00		40.00
73090	Forearm X ray, AP and lateral	50.00	1	50.00		50.00
73600	Ankle X ray, AP and lateral	50.00	1	50.00	0.00	50.00
82465	Cholesterol test	30.00	1	30.00		30.00
82947	Glucose—quantitative	60.00	2	30.00		60.00
83718	HDL cholesterol test	25.00	1	25.00		25.00
85022	CBC w/ diff	10.00	1	10.00		10.00
90703	Tetanus injection	20.00	1	20.00		20.00
90782	Injection	180.00	6	30.00		180.00
93000	Electroencephalogram—EEG	120.00	2	60.00		120.00
93015	Treadmill stress test	300.00	2	150.00		300.00
99201	OF—New patient, focused	140.00	1	140.00		140.00
99203	OF—New patient, complete physical	200.00	1	200.00		200.00
99204	OF—New patient, mod. complex	100.00	1	100.00		100.00
99211	OF—Established patient, minimal	150.00	3	50.00		150.00
99212	OF—Established patient, focused	1987.00	17	116.88		1987.00
99213	OF—Established patient, expanded	396.00	3	132.00		396.00
99214	OF—Established patient, routine exam	240.00	3	80.00		240.00
99215	OF—Established patient, complex	100.00	1	100.00		100.00
Z9070	MMR	18.00	1	18.00		18.00

Total Procedure Charges	$4,291.00
Total Product Charges	$0.00
Total Inside Lab Charges	$0.00
Total Outside Lab Charges	$0.00
Total Insurance Payments	-$702.50
Total Cash Co-payments	$0.00
Total Check Co-payments	$0.00
Total Credit Card Co-payments	$0.00
Total Patient Cash Payments	-$70.00
Total Patient Check Payments	-$205.00
Total Credit Card Payments	$0.00
Total Deductibles	$0.00
Total Debit Adjustments	$0.00
Total Credit Adjustments	$0.00
Total Medicare Debit Adjustments	$0.00
Total Medicare Credit Adjustments	$0.00
Net Effect on Accounts Receivable	$3,313.50

Figure 6-3 *Practice Analysis Report*

you could print a report for a specific time period. These options let you customize the report to display only the data you need.

4. In the *Date From Range* box, the current date appears as the default. Enter the program date **9/4/98** in this box.

5. Zoom the report and review the information shown for the Family Care Center's patients.

6. Print the report and then close the Preview Report window.

7. Display the Patient Aging report and review the information provided. Do not print this report, unless instructed otherwise.

8. Display the Practice Analysis report. The program date should be entered to replace the current date.

PATIENT STATEMENTS

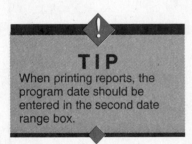

TIP

When printing reports, the program date should be entered in the second date range box.

Printing patient statements is a straightforward process with the *MediSoft* software. A **patient statement** shows the services rendered to a patient, total payments, total charges, adjustments, and the balance due. (See Figure 6-4 on page 121.) Usually, you will print patient statements at the end of each month and then mail them to patients.

After printing patient statements, the *MediSoft* program automatically updates the patient data file so that the next time you print patient statements, only the new procedure charges will appear. The old transactions will not be shown on next month's statements.

As you will learn in the next section, you can customize many of the *MediSoft* reports. You could, for example, print a message on each statement. Or, you could customize the statements to print on pre-printed forms.

PRACTICE EXERCISE 6-3

Printing Patient Statements

1. Select *Patient Statements* from the Reports menu.

2. Highlight the *Patient Statement* option in the Open Report dialog box and then click the **OK** button.

3. Choose to view the report on the screen.

4. Enter **BAREL000** in both of the *Chart Number Range* fields to print a patient statement for Ellen Barmenstein only. Then, click the **OK** button.

5. Enter **8/1/98** and **9/4/98** in the *Date From Range* boxes.

Family Care Center
285 Stephenson Boulevard
Stephenson, OH 60089
(614)555-0100

Statement Date
9/4/98

Page
1

Ellen Barmenstein
1774 Grand Street
Stephenson, OH 60089

Account Number
BAREL000

Date	Document	Description	Case Number	Amount
		Previous Balance		**0.00**
8/28/98	9808280000	OF—Established patient, focused	1	60.00
8/28/98	9808280000	Patient payment, cash	1	-20.00
9/4/98	9809040000	Insurance Company, payment	1	-40.00
9/4/98	9809040000	OF—Established patient, routine exam	29	80.00

Total Payments	Total Charges	Total Adjustments	Balance Due
-$60.00	$140.00	$0.00	**$80.00**

Figure 6-4 *Patient Statement*

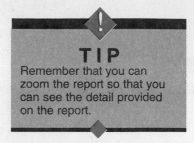

6. Review the patient statement.

7. Print the report, but make sure that this report includes only one statement.

LIST REPORTS

As you are aware, *MediSoft* stores most of the data for a medical practice in various lists. There are procedure lists, diagnosis lists, patient lists, insurance carrier lists, and so on. You can use the *Custom Report List* option to access the list reports.

PRACTICE EXERCISE 6-4

Viewing List Reports

1. Pull down the **Reports** menu and choose *Custom Report List*.

2. Click on the **List** radio button in the Open Report dialog box to show only the list reports. (See Figure 6-5.)

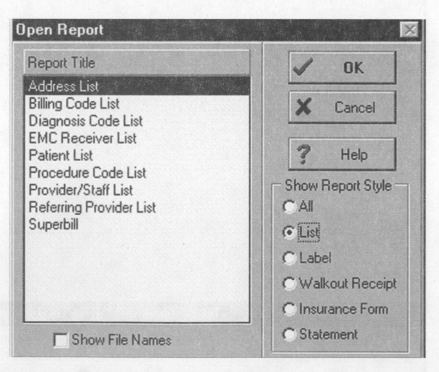

Figure 6-5 *Open Report Dialog Box with Lists*

3. Select the *Procedure Code List* and then click the **OK** button.

4. Choose to display the list on the screen.

5. Review the procedures shown on the report.

6. Display a patient list.

7. Display any of the other lists if you are interested in the information they contain.

DESIGNING CUSTOM REPORTS AND BILLS ◆

You can generate numerous reports using the *MediSoft* program. However, there may be situations when you want to customize a report to meet a particular need. For example, you could design a special report to be sent to an insurance carrier. In these instances, you can use the *MediSoft* Report Designer to modify an existing report or create a completely new report. This very powerful tool provides all the features you need to prepare a new report layout.

Although this tutorial does not cover the Report Designer, you can explore this option on your own. To access the Report Designer, choose the *Design Custom Reports and Bills* option from the Reports menu. Remember that you can use the help system to learn more about the Report Designer if you have any questions.

CHECKPOINT

1. Which report shows each patient and identifies each account as current or past due?

   Patient Ledger

2. Which report shows the total revenue for each procedure?

   The Practice Analysis

3. Which report lists all of the procedure codes?

   Procedure Day Sheet

4. Which report includes information organized by patient and is typically printed at the end of each day?

   Day Sheet (Patient)

5. Which option would allow you to create a patient statement that can be output to a pre-printed form?

   Printing Analysis

PRACTICE EXERCISE 6-5

Exiting the Program

Practice quitting the software by following the steps listed below.

1. Choose *Exit* from the File menu or use the toolbar to select this option.

2. Click the **Exit Program** button in the Backup Reminder window. Do **NOT** choose the backup option.

3. Store your disks in a safe place. You do not have to make a backup copy of your data disk since you did not enter any new data during this session.

Chapter

6

CHAPTER REVIEW

DEFINE THE TERMS

Write a definition for each term: (Obj. 6-1)

1. Aging

   Pg 113

   _____

   _____

   _____

2. Receivables

   Pg 114

   _____

   _____

   _____

   _____

3. Cash flow

   Pg 114

   _____

   _____

   _____

   _____

4. Payables

   Pg 114

   _____

   _____

   _____

   _____

Chapter 6 ◆ *Producing Reports and Patient Statements*

CHECK YOUR UNDERSTANDING

5. What information is included on the Practice Analysis report? *(Obj. 6-6)*

    Pg 117

    _____

    _____

    _____

6. Does the *MediSoft* program let you set up filters to print only selected information on a report? Explain. *(Obj. 6-2)*

    _____

    _____

    _____

    _____

    _____

7. Describe how you can use the controls in the Preview Report window to review the information on a report. *(Obj. 6-2)*

    Pg 115

    _____

    _____

    _____

    _____

8. What information is included on the Patient Ledger report? *(Obj. 6-4)*

    Pg 117

    _____

    _____

    _____

    _____

9. List several reasons why you might need to use the *MediSoft* Report Designer to customize a report. *(Obj. 6-10)*

Pg 123

_____

_____

_____

_____

 THINK IT THROUGH

10. Why is the information on a Patient Aging report or a Primary Insurance Aging report so valuable in monitoring accounts receivable data? *(Objs. 6-5, 6-7)*

_____

_____

_____

_____

_____

_____

_____

_____

_____

_____

_____

_____

PROCESSING CLAIMS

WHAT YOU NEED TO KNOW

To complete this chapter, you need to know how to:

◆ Enter information in *MediSoft*.

◆ Navigate the *MediSoft* software.

◆ Search for information in a *MediSoft* database.

◆ Enter patient and case information.

◆ Record procedure charges and payments.

◆ Print reports.

WHAT YOU WILL LEARN

When you finish this chapter, you will be able to:

1. Define the terms introduced in this chapter.

2. Describe the claim management process.

3. Create claims.

4. Edit claim information.

5. Print HCFA-1500 claim forms.

6. Explain how to mark and delete claims.

7. Print a Primary Insurance Aging report.

KEY TERMS

EMC receiver   (Electronic Media Claims) An insurance company or a clearing-house set up to electronically receive and process claims for medical practices.

National Data Corporation (NDC)   A company that serves as a clearinghouse through which you can send electronic claims via the *MediSoft* program.

Status   The current disposition of a medical claim.

CLAIM MANAGEMENT

Claim management is an important activity in the patient billing process. Processing claims involves creating claims, editing them (if necessary), and sending the claims to the various insurance companies for payment. Claims can be sent electronically or on paper, and the *MediSoft* program can accommodate either method. In this tutorial, however, you will focus on processing claims on paper.

Depending on the medical practice, a billing assistant may process claims daily, weekly, or monthly. The Family Care Center processes paper claims on a daily basis. As you work through this chapter, you will learn how to process claims. You will also print a Primary Insurance Aging report that you can use to track claims sent to insurance carriers.

To process claims, you will use the *Claim Management* option in the Activities menu. When you select this option, *MediSoft* displays the Claim Management window as shown in Figure 7-1 on page 131. As you can see, this window includes options to edit, create, print/send, and delete claims. You will learn how to use each of these options in the following sections.

As you use the *MediSoft* program, the list of claims in the Claim Management window will continue to expand. Each day you will add new claims to the list of those that have already been sent. Some claims may be marked as challenged or rejected while others may be held for processing. Then, from time to time, you can remove or delete some claims after you no longer need the claims information.

Creating Claims

After you enter procedure charges, the next step is to create the insurance claim forms. The *MediSoft* program simplifies this task by automating many aspects of this process. In a previous chapter, you learned that you can create a claim immediately after you record a procedure charge transaction. In this chapter, you will learn that you can also use the Claim Management features to process claims in batches.

Using the Claim Management capabilities, you can create claims for all procedure charges or you can direct the program to create claims that match certain criteria. For example, you can create claims for all

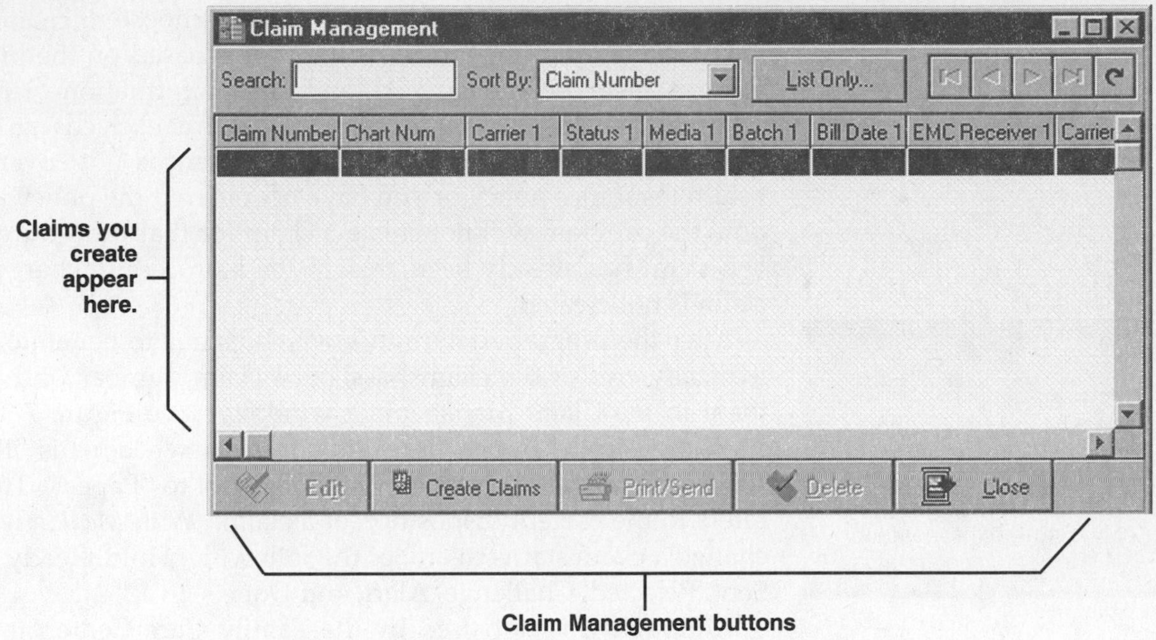

Claims you create appear here.

Claim Management buttons

Figure 7-1 *Claim Management Window*

charges entered on a certain date. Or, you can have the program create claims only for a specific insurance carrier. These options and others are available in the Create Claims window. (See Figure 7-2 below.)

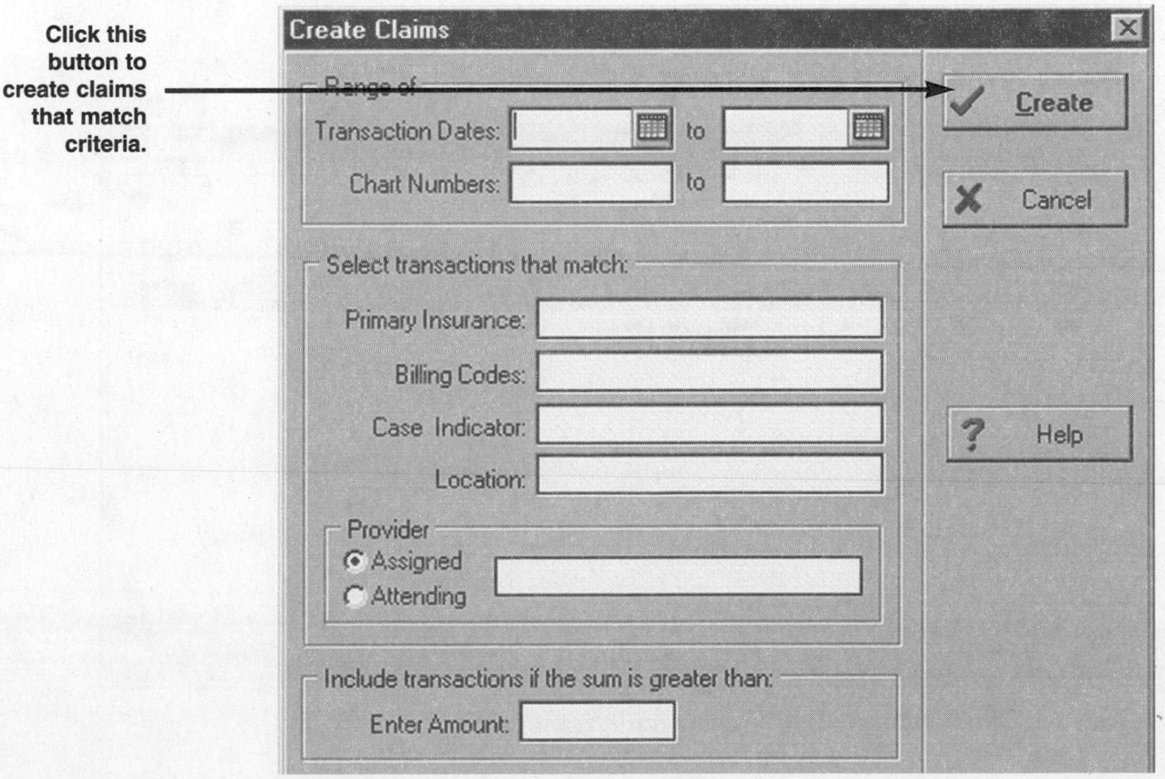

Click this button to create claims that match criteria.

Figure 7-2 *Create Claims Window*

After you enter your search criteria and choose to create claims, the *MediSoft* program generates the claims based on the procedure charges, insurance policy data, and other information you entered for each case. The *MediSoft* application looks at each charge to determine if it should create a claim. If a patient is not covered by a health insurance policy or you have not entered the policy information, the program will not create a claim for that procedure charge. If a claim has already been created for a procedure charge, a new claim is not created.

After the program determines which claims to generate, it automatically creates the claims, assigns a claim number, and displays them in the Claim Management window. (See Figure 7-3 below.) As shown in the figure, the status of the new claims is "Ready to send" and the billing method or media is set to "Paper." The **status** refers to the current disposition of a claim. With *MediSoft*, you can change a claim status to any of the following: Hold, Ready to send, Sent, Rejected, Challenge, Alert, and Done.

Although it is not used by the Family Care Center, the Claim Management window includes a column to show the EMC receiver. An **EMC receiver** is an insurance company or clearinghouse set up to electronically receive and process medical claims submitted by the medical practice. An EMC receiver is needed to process claims electronically.

> **!**
>
> **TIP**
>
> The *Status* column is not wide enough to show the complete message in some instances. For example, only "Ready to" appears for the "Ready to send" status.

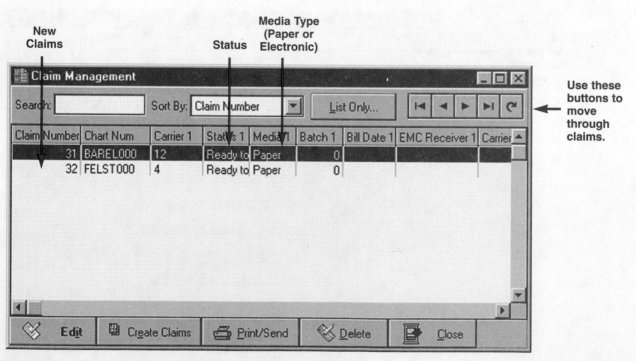

Figure 7-3 *Claim Management Window with New Claims*

PRACTICE EXERCISE 7-1

Creating Claims

The Family Care Center processes new claims every day. Follow the steps provided below to create the insurance claims for the transactions that you entered on September 4, 1998.

1. Start the *MediSoft* program.

2. Set the program date to **9/4/98**.

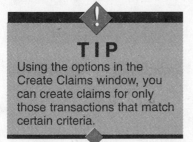

TIP

Using the options in the Create Claims window, you can create claims for only those transactions that match certain criteria.

3. Pull down the **Activities** menu and choose the *Claim Management* option to display the Claim Management window.

4. Click the **Create Claims** button to display the window that lets you specify which claims to create.

5. Enter **9/4/98** in both of the *Range of Transaction Dates* fields so that the program will create the claims for that date only.

6. Click the **Create** button in the Create Claims window to generate the claims for the transactions recorded on September 4, 1998.

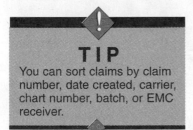

TIP

You can sort claims by claim number, date created, carrier, chart number, batch, or EMC receiver.

7. In the Claim Management window, choose **Carrier 1** in the *Sort By* field to sort the claims by insurance company.

8. Compare the claims listed on your screen to those shown in Figure 7-4. Verify that all of the claims are marked as "Ready to send" and the media is set to "Paper."

Claim Number	Chart Num	Carrier 1	Status 1	Media 1	Batch 1	Bill Date 1	EMC Receiver 1	Carrier
5	WONJO000	1	Ready to	Paper	0			
6	WONLI000	1	Ready to	Paper	0			
1	BAREL000	12	Ready to	Paper	0			
2	LOMCE000	4	Ready to	Paper	0			8
3	LOMLI000	4	Ready to	Paper	0			8
4	SMOJI000	8	Ready to	Paper	0			

Search: | Sort By: Carrier 1 | List Only... | Edit | Create Claims | Print/Send | Delete | Close

Figure 7-4 *Claim Management (September 4, Claims)*

Editing Claims

You can edit any of the claims that appear in the Claim Management window. Although the claim information generated by the *MediSoft* program is usually correct, you may have a reason to change some of this information. For example, you could change the status for a specific claim from "Sent" to "Ready to send" if you need to reprint a specific claim. Or, you could select a different insurance carrier if this information was incorrectly recorded in a patient's case.

Simply highlight a claim and click the **Edit** button to edit the corresponding information. When you choose to edit a claim, the *MediSoft* program displays the Edit Claim window as shown in Figure 7-5 below. As you can see, you can change the claim status, billing method, billing date, insurance carrier, or EMC receiver for any of the three carriers. Using this option, you can also view the transactions associated with a claim or attach a comment.

Edit claim folders. →

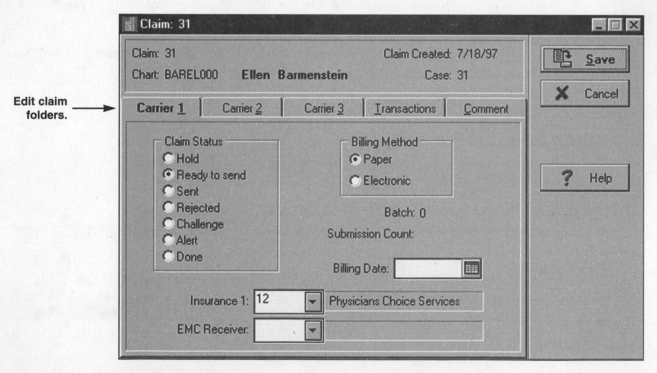

Figure 7-5 *Edit Claim Window*

PRACTICE EXERCISE 7-2

Editing Claims

Follow the steps listed here to learn how you can review and edit the information stored for a claim.

1. Select (highlight) any one of the claims shown in the Claim Management window.

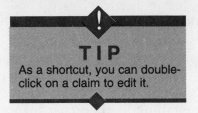
2. Click the **Edit** button to view/update the claim you chose.

3. Review the information in the *Carrier 1*, *Carrier 2*, and *Carrier 3* folders, but do not change any of the data.

4. Review the transaction data.

5. Enter the following note in the *Comment* folder: **Claim sent, but approval pending due to change in patient status**.

6. Save the change you made to the claim.

Proofing Claims Using the List Only Option

As the list of previously sent claims grows, it can be difficult to verify the new claims to be sent. The *List Only* feature is useful in proofing new claims. You can use this option to list only those claims created on a certain date or choose to view claims to be sent to a specific carrier. After you use this option, you should always select it again and reset the criteria to the defaults so that all of the claims appear in the Claim Management window.

PRACTICE EXERCISE 7-3

Reviewing Insurance Claims

Learn how to use the *List Only* option to review insurance claims before you send them. Follow the steps provided here.

1. In the Claim Management window, click the **List Only** button.

2. Enter **Physicians Choice Services** in the *Insurance Carrier* field and click the **Apply** button.

 You should see only those claims that match the criteria you set. However, you could have selected several different criteria to fine-tune your search.

3. Before you continue, you need to reset the *List Only* options so that all of the claims appear. Click the **List Only** button again to display the List Only Claims That Match window. Click the **Defaults** button to reset all of the options and then click the **Apply** button.

4. Verify that all of the claims appear in the list.

Printing Insurance Claim Forms

After creating new claims and proofing them, you are ready to print/send the claims. The Family Care Center prints its claims using the HCFA-1500 (Primary) form and then mails the completed insurance forms to the insurance carriers. However, this entire process could be handled electronically if the medical practice was set up accordingly.

To print or send the new claims, you will use the **Print/Send** button. The program asks you to select the billing method (paper or electronic). If you are printing the claim forms, you must select the appropriate HCFA report format. Although there are several different HCFA report options from which to choose, some of them have minor variations that are required to accommodate different printers. Other HCFA report options are available to process Medicare claims. For our purposes, you should always use the HCFA-1500 (Primary) report.

When you preview a report or print the final claim forms, the data do not seem to be formatted properly. Remember that a medical office must print the claims on blank HCFA-1500 forms and send the completed forms to the respective insurance carriers. The location of the data corresponds to the required fields on the form. A completed HCFA-1500 form is shown in Figure 7-6 on page 137.

> **IMPORTANT:** The *MediSoft* program changes the claim status from "Ready to send" to "Sent" only after you actually print the claims. If you don't want to waste paper printing the claim forms, you can print them to a file or manually mark the claims as "Sent."

PRACTICE EXERCISE 7-4

Printing Insurance Claims

After you create the insurance claims, the next step is to print or electronically send them. Follow the instructions provided below to print insurance claim forms.

1. Click the **Print/Send** button in the Claim Management window.

2. Make sure that you have selected the option to print claims using the paper billing method. Click the **OK** button to continue.

3. In the Open Report window, choose the **HCFA 1500 (Primary)** report and click the **OK** button.

4. Choose to preview the reports on the screen.

5. Accept the default settings in the Data Selection Questions window.

6. Review the claim reports.

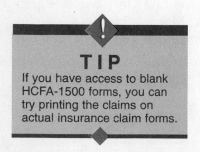

TIP

If you have access to blank HCFA-1500 forms, you can try printing the claims on actual insurance claim forms.

PLEASE
DO NOT
STAPLE
IN THIS
AREA

PHYSICIANS CHOICE SERVICES
900 BLUE ROCK TURNPIKE
CLARKSVILLE, OH 60817

CARRIER →

| | PICA | **HEALTH INSURANCE CLAIM FORM** | PICA | |

1. MEDICARE	MEDICAID	CHAMPUS	CHAMPVA	GROUP HEALTH PLAN	FECA BLK LUNG	OTHER	1a. INSURED'S I.D. NUMBER	(FOR PROGRAM IN ITEM 1)
(Medicare#)	(Medicaid #)	(Sponsor's SSN)	(VA File #)	(SSN or ID)	(SSN) X	(ID)	13056	

2. PATIENT'S NAME (Last Name, First Name, Middle Initial)	3. PATIENT'S BIRTH DATE / SEX	4. INSURED'S NAME (Last Name, First Name, Middle Initial)
BARMENSTEIN ELLEN	MM 10 DD 16 YY 71 M☐ F☒	BARMENSTEIN ELLEN

5. PATIENT'S ADDRESS (No., Street)	6. PATIENT RELATIONSHIP TO INSURED	7. INSURED'S ADDRESS (No., Street)
1774 GRAND STREET	Self X Spouse☐ Child☐ Other☐	1774 GRAND STREET

| CITY: STEPHENSON | STATE: OH | 8. PATIENT STATUS | CITY: STEPHENSON | STATE: OH |

| ZIP CODE: 60089 | TELEPHONE (Include Area Code): (614) 274 4242 | Single☐ Married☐ Other☐ | ZIP CODE: 60817 | TELEPHONE (INCLUDE AREA CODE): (614) 274 4242 |

9. OTHER INSURED'S NAME (Last Name, First Name, Middle Initial)	10. IS PATIENT'S CONDITION RELATED TO:	11. INSURED'S POLICY GROUP OR FECA NUMBER
BARMENSTEIN ELLEN		K1047

Employed X Full-Time Student☐ Part-Time Student☐

| a. OTHER INSURED'S POLICY OR GROUP NUMBER | a. EMPLOYMENT? (CURRENT OR PREVIOUS) YES☐ NO☐ | a. INSURED'S DATE OF BIRTH MM 10 DD 16 YY 71 M☐ F☒ SEX |

| b. OTHER INSURED'S DATE OF BIRTH MM 10 DD 16 YY 71 M☐ F☒ SEX | b. AUTO ACCIDENT? YES☐ NO X PLACE (State) | b. EMPLOYER'S NAME OR SCHOOL NAME: SARA'S DRESSES |

| c. EMPLOYER'S NAME OR SCHOOL NAME: SARA'S DRESSES | c. OTHER ACCIDENT? YES☐ NO☐ | c. INSURANCE PLAN NAME OR PROGRAM NAME: PHYSICIANS CHOICE SERVICES |

| d. INSURANCE PLAN NAME OR PROGRAM NAME: MEDICARE | 10d. RESERVED FOR LOCAL USE | d. IS THERE ANOTHER HEALTH BENEFIT PLAN? YES☐ NO X *If yes*, return to and complete item 9 a-d. |

READ BACK OF FORM BEFORE COMPLETING & SIGNING THIS FORM.

12. PATIENT'S OR AUTHORIZED PERSON'S SIGNATURE I authorize the release of any medical or other information necessary to process this claim. I also request payment of government benefits either to myself or to the party who accepts assignment below.

SIGNED _SIGNATURE ON FILE_ DATE _7/18/98_

13. INSURED'S OR AUTHORIZED PERSON'S SIGNATURE I authorize payment of medical benefits to the undersigned physician or supplier for services described below.

SIGNED _SIGNATURE ON FILE_

PATIENT AND INSURED INFORMATION

| 14. DATE OF CURRENT: ◄ ILLNESS (First symptom) OR INJURY (Accident) OR PREGNANCY (LMP) | 15. IF PATIENT HAS HAD SAME OR SIMILAR ILLNESS. GIVE FIRST DATE MM DD YY | 16. DATES PATIENT UNABLE TO WORK IN CURRENT OCCUPATION FROM MM DD YY TO MM DD YY |

| 17. NAME OF REFERRING PHYSICIAN OR OTHER SOURCE | 17a. I.D. NUMBER OF REFERRING PHYSICIAN | 18. HOSPITALIZATION DATES RELATED TO CURRENT SERVICES FROM MM DD YY TO MM DD YY |

| 19. RESERVED FOR LOCAL USE | 20. OUTSIDE LAB? YES☐ NO X $ CHARGES |

21. DIAGNOSIS OR NATURE OF ILLNESS OR INJURY. (RELATE ITEMS 1,2,3 OR 4 TO ITEM 24E BY LINE)

1. V70.0   3.

2.   4.

22. MEDICAID RESUBMISSION CODE   ORIGINAL REF. NO.

23. PRIOR AUTHORIZATION NUMBER

24. A. DATE(S) OF SERVICE From MM DD YY To MM DD YY	B. Place of Service	C. Type of Service	D. PROCEDURES, SERVICES, OR SUPPLIES (Explain Unusual Circumstances) CPT/HCPCS MODIFIER	E. DIAGNOSIS CODE	F. $ CHARGES	G. DAYS OR UNITS	H. EPSDT Family Plan	I. EMG	J. COB	K. RESERVED FOR LOCAL USE
1	9 4 98 9 4 98	11	5	82465	1	30.00	1				60-3872-8
2	9 4 98 9 4 98	11	1	82947	1	30.00	1				60-3872-8
3											
4											
5											
6											

25. FEDERAL TAX I.D. NUMBER SSN EIN	26. PATIENT'S ACCOUNT NO.	27. ACCEPT ASSIGNMENT? (For govt. claims, see back)	28. TOTAL CHARGE	29. AMOUNT PAID	30. BALANCE DUE
810-99-1110 X	BAREL000	YES X NO☐	$ 60.00	$	$ 60.00

31. SIGNATURE OF PHYSICIAN OR SUPPLIER INCLUDING DEGREES OR CREDENTIALS (I certify that the statements on the reverse apply to this bill and are made a part thereof.)

SIGNED _7/18/98_ DATE

32. NAME AND ADDRESS OF FACILITY WHERE SERVICES WERE RENDERED (If other than home or office)

DR. MARION DAVIS
3500 MAIN STREET
STEPHENSON, OH 60092

33. PHYSICIAN'S, SUPPLIER'S BILLING NAME, ADDRESS, ZIP CODE & PHONE #

FAMILY CARE CENTER
285 STEPHENSON BOULEVARD
STEPHENSON, OH 60089
PIN# 60-3872-8   GRP#

PHYSICIAN OR SUPPLIER INFORMATION

(APPROVED BY AMA COUNCIL ON MEDICAL SERVICE 8/88)
WHCFA-1500-1-90

PLEASE PRINT OR TYPE

FORM HCFA-1500   (12-90)
FORM OWCP-1500   FORM RRB-1500

Figure 7-6 *Completed HCFA-1500 Form*

7. Print the claims unless you are instructed otherwise.

8. Close the report window.

9. Review the status for the claims.

10. If you did not actually print the claims, you must manually mark each claim as "Sent." Edit each claim and change the claim status to indicate that you sent the claims.

11. Close the Claim Management window.

Marking Accepted Claims

When you print or send claims, the software automatically changes the status to "Sent." If you send claims electronically and a link is established to receive an audit report, the software can also be set up to mark whether a claim was accepted, challenged, or rejected. This functionality, however, requires that you send claims electronically through the National Data Corporation. **National Data Corporation (NDC)** is a clearinghouse through which you can send electronic claims via the *MediSoft* program. For this tutorial, processing electronic claims is only discussed, not actually practiced.

If you need to manually mark a claim, you can edit it and change the status by choosing the appropriate claim status. You may, for example, need to change the status of a claim from "Rejected" to "Hold."

Deleting Claims

Using the Claim Management functions, you can delete claims that are no longer needed so that the list of claims is more manageable. Although many medical practices leave "sent" claims active for quite some time, you can remove the old claims that have been sent and paid by the insurance carriers. For our purposes, you should not need to delete any claims that you create.

What if you accidentally create claims that should not be included in the list? Rather than deleting the claims, you could mark them as "Hold." This method is preferable to deleting the claims.

C H E C K P O I N T

1. Which option from the application menu do you select to access the claim management functions?

Pg 130

2. Using the Claim Management window, which button lets you create new claims?

_Pg 131_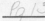

3. What status is assigned to a claim before it is printed or sent?

_Pg 136_

4. After claims are printed, what status does the program use to mark those claims?

_Pg 136_

5. Which form do you use to process claims on paper?

_Pg 136_   HFCA

INSURANCE CARRIER ANALYSIS

As you learned in the previous chapter, the insurance aging reports include information that lets you review the current insurance claims. Using the Primary Insurance Aging report, for example, you can analyze which of the primary carriers process claims promptly and which are slow to pay. As shown on Figure 7-7, page 141, the entire procedure charge appears for each claim even though an insurance company may cover only a portion of any one claim.

The *MediSoft* program automatically updates the information that appears on the insurance aging reports. When you send claims either electronically or on paper, the program adds those claims to the list of outstanding claims. The program removes a claim from the aging report when you post an insurance payment transaction to the corresponding procedure charge.

PRACTICE EXERCISE 7-5

Printing an Insurance Aging Report

Print an insurance aging report to review the insurance claims you just sent. Follow the steps provided here.

1. Select the *Primary Insurance Aging* option from the Reports menu.

2. Choose to display the report on your screen.

3. Leave the Data Selection Questions blank.

4. Review the information contained on the report and then print it.

5. Close the report window.

6. Exit the program if you are finished for this session.

7. Back up your data disk.

Family Care Center Primary Insurance Aging						
Date of Service	Procedure	–Past– 0-30	–Past– 31-60	–Past– 61-90	–Past– 91-999	Total Balance
Medicare (1)						(215)599-0205
WONJO000	**Jo Wong**					
9/4/98	99212	60.00				60.00
9/4/98	85022	10.00				10.00
Claim5	Billed: 9/4/98	70.00	0.00	0.00	0.00	70.00
WONLI000	**Li Yu Wong**					
9/4/98	99211	50.00				50.00
Claim6	Billed: 9/4/98	50.00	0.00	0.00	0.00	50.00
	Insurance Totals	$120.00	$0.00	$0.00	$0.00	$120.00
Physicians Choice Services (12)						(614)843-8872
BAREL000	**Ellen Barmenstein**					
9/4/98	99214	80.00				80.00
Claim1	Billed: 9/4/98	80.00	0.00	0.00	0.00	80.00
	Insurance Totals	$80.00	$0.00	$0.00	$0.00	$80.00
Blue Cross/Blue Shield (4)						(614)241-9000
LOMCE000	**Cedera Lomos**					
9/4/98	99204	100.00				100.00
Claim2	Billed: 9/4/98	100.00	0.00	0.00	0.00	100.00
LOMLI000	**LIsa Lomos**					
9/4/98	99203	200.00				200.00
9/4/98	Z9070	18.00				18.00
Claim3	Billed: 9/4/98	218.00	0.00	0.00	0.00	218.00
	Insurance Totals	$318.00	$0.00	$0.00	$0.00	$318.00
Physician Alliance of Ohio (8)						(514)929-0320
SMOJI000	**Jim Smolowski**					
9/4/98	99214	80.00				80.00
9/4/98	82947	30.00				30.00
9/4/98	93000	60.00				60.00
Claim4	Billed: 9/4/98	170.00	0.00	0.00	0.00	170.00
	Insurance Totals	$170.00	$0.00	$0.00	$0.00	$170.00

Figure 7-7 *Primary Insurance Aging Claim Report*

Name _____   **Date** _____

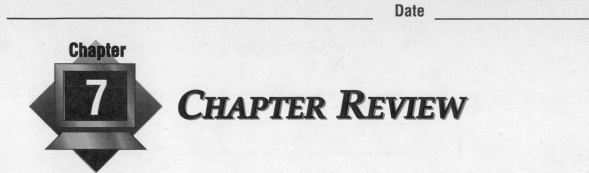

Chapter

7

CHAPTER REVIEW

DEFINE THE TERMS

Write a definition for each term: *(Obj. 7-1)*

1. Status

   Pg 130
   _____

   _____

2. NDC

   _____

   _____

3. EMC receiver

   _____

   _____

   _____

CHECK YOUR UNDERSTANDING

4. What status does the program assign to new claims it creates? What other status options are used by the program? *(Obj. 7-1)*

    Pg 132 b
   _____

   _____

   _____

   _____

   _____

   _____

5. What steps are required to print new claims that you already created? (Objs. 7-2, 4, & 5)

Pg 135

_____

_____

_____

_____

_____

6. What information is provided on the insurance aging reports? How would you use this information? (Obj. 7-7)

Pg 189

_____

_____

_____

_____

_____

7. Can you edit claims after you create them? Why might you need to edit a claim? (Obj. 7-4)

Pg 134

_____

_____

_____

_____

8. When does the *MediSoft* program automatically mark claims to indicate that they were sent? (Objs. 7-2, 5)

Pg 138

_____

_____

_____

_____

9. Why would you use the option to delete a claim? *(Obj. 7-6)*

_Pg 138_

_____

_____

_____

 THINK IT THROUGH

10. List the steps to create and process claims. *(Obj. 7-2)*

_____

_____

_____

_____

_____

_____

_____

_____

_____

_____

_____

_____

_____

_____

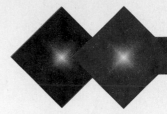

Now that you have completed the tutorial, you are ready to begin the patient billing simulation using the *MediSoft* program. As the new billing assistant for the Family Care Center, your job is to process the patient billing for the medical practice. The simulation takes place from Tuesday, September 8, 1998 through Friday, September 11, 1998. Work begins on Tuesday, since Monday, September 7 is Labor Day.

As you complete the simulation, you may notice that the volume of work is not the same as you would expect in an actual medical practice. However, the tasks you will perform are similar to those a billing assistant would perform on a daily basis.

Before you begin, review the Office Procedures Manual shown on pages 148 through 150. Then, refer to the step-by-step instructions provided on pages 151-156 to complete the simulation. If you need assistance using the software, refer to the tutorial or use the Help information built into the software.

Family

Care

Center

~

A Patient

Billing

Simulation

Office Procedures Manual

Review the office procedures for the Family Care Center. Some of these tasks are already completed for you, but in an actual office, you would perform each of these duties.

DAILY TASKS BEFORE PATIENTS ARRIVE

- ◆ Assist receptionist in completing a superbill for each patient with a scheduled appointment. Fill in the patient's name, address, chart number, and the date.

- ◆ Gather the materials for the day: *MediSoft* data disk, yesterday afternoon's superbills, and any receipts (cash or checks) from the previous day. The receptionist keeps the receipts in a locked drawer overnight.

- ◆ Prepare a change fund for the receptionist.

- ◆ Turn on the computer and start *MediSoft*.

MORNING TASKS

Each morning you must enter the transactions and payments from the previous afternoon, and then prepare a bank deposit slip. Deposits are usually made at noon.

- ◆ Enter the superbill data from the previous afternoon.

- ◆ If necessary, update any patient accounts.

- ◆ Open the mail and record each check received. Enter the payment amount and the check number. Indicate whether the payment is from an insurer or a patient.

- Prepare a bank deposit slip for the checks received in the mail and for receipts on hand from the previous day.

- Print a Patient Day Sheet and Procedure Day Sheet for the previous day. Use the day sheets to check the accuracy of the bank deposit.

- Give the day sheets to the office manager and take the deposit to the bank.

AFTERNOON TASKS ◆

During the afternoon, your primary task is to enter the patient information, charges, and payments for those patients who had morning appointments. Other tasks include printing claim forms for the previous day's transactions.

- Create, print, and mail the insurance claim forms for the previous day's visits.

- Gather the Patient Information Forms for the new patients who had morning appointments, and enter this information into the system.

- Update any information for established patients.

- Using the superbills provided by the receptionist, enter the data for patients seen in the morning.

- Time permitting, enter the transactions for the afternoon appointments.

- Back up the patient billing data.

OTHER TASKS DURING THE DAY ◆

- Respond to calls from patients about their accounts.

- Relieve the receptionist when needed.

- Make collection calls to patients and insurers.

- Call insurers about managed-care cases as needed.

- Fill out (or print) special forms for disability and so forth.

WEEKLY TASKS ◆

- Since there are no appointments scheduled on Thursday afternoons, print a Patient Aging report and consult with the office manager regarding any overdue accounts. If necessary, contact any patients or insurance carriers concerning past due account balances. Write off bad debts after consulting with the office manager. (Typically, these are for charges more than a year old where there is no chance of collecting from the patient or insurer.)

◆ On Friday mornings, prepare the appropriate patient statements:

   1st Friday—Patients A-F
   2nd Friday—Patients G-L
   3rd Friday—Patients M-R
   4th Friday—Patients S-Z
   5th Friday (if there is one)—Skip

◆ Print a Practice Analysis report.

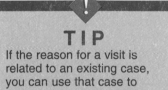

Step-by-Step Instructions

TUESDAY, SEPTEMBER 8, 1998

1. Remove Source Documents 15 through 26 on pages 187-210. Review the information provided on the source documents before entering data.

2. Start the *MediSoft* program.

3. Set the program date to **September 4, 1998.** The patient transactions from Friday afternoon, September 4, have not been recorded yet. **Note:** The office was closed on Monday, September 7 for Labor Day.

4. Record these transactions from last Friday using the information provided on Source Documents 15-18. Use the *Enter Transactions* option to record the procedure charges and payments. Print a walkout receipt for each patient.

   ◆ Use the superbill for Janine Bell (Source Document 15) to record the procedure charge and payment. Janine is covered by her husband's policy from U.S. Life (Policy #: 50632, Group #: 6209). The policy provides 80% coverage with a $200 deductible. Remember to enter **09/04/98** for the transaction date and print a walkout receipt.

   ◆ Enter the information to record the procedure charge for Felix Suarez (Source Document 16). The patient made no payment. Create a new case for this office visit. You will need to review an earlier case to get the necessary policy information. Or, you can copy the existing case, and then change the description and diagnosis.

   ◆ Record the two procedure charges and payment written on Sarah Fitzwilliams's superbill (Source Document 17). Sarah is covered by her father's Champ VA insurance (Policy #: 457091, Group #: 3265). The policy pays 80% of covered procedures.

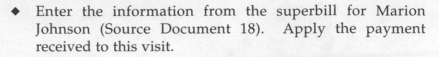

♦ Enter the information from the superbill for Marion Johnson (Source Document 18). Apply the payment received to this visit.

5. Four checks that were received last Friday have not been processed. The information you need to record these payments is provided on Source Document 19. Enter these payment transactions. Be sure that the program date is set to 9/4/98.

6. Print a Patient Day Sheet and a Procedure Day Sheet for Friday, September 4, 1998.

7. Verify that you have entered the information correctly. The total cash and checks on hand should be $1,480.50. Does this amount equal the sum of the payments shown on the day sheet for Friday, September 4? If the amounts match, continue with the next step. Otherwise, find your error, correct it, and print updated reports. After verifying the amounts, you would complete a bank deposit slip and take the deposit to the bank.

8. Create the insurance claim forms for the patient charges you just entered. Use 09/04/98 to create claim forms for that date only. Print the claims using the HCFA-1500 (primary) form. After you have printed and proofed them, you would mail these forms to the corresponding insurance companies.

9. Change the program date to **September 8, 1998** since you will now begin entering some of today's transactions.

10. Set up patient accounts for two patients who had appointments with Dr. Yan this morning. Since Mr. and Mrs. Andrews have not had appointments since the practice began using *MediSoft*, they will need to be entered as if they were new patients. Use the Patient Information Forms shown in Source Documents 20 and 21 to record the patient information.

11. Update the patient information for James Smith (Source Document 22).

12. Enter the procedure charges and payments for the patients who had appointments this morning—Darla Andrews, Bill Andrews, Cedera Lomos, and Stanley Feldman (Source Documents 23-26). Print a walkout receipt for each patient. Be sure that the program date is set to Tuesday (09/08/98) when you record the transactions.

   Notes: (a) Use the existing case for Cedera Lomos since the reason for this visit is the same as the last visit. (b) Create a new case for Stanley Feldman's visit. He does not have health insurance. Apply his payment to this new case.

13. Exit the *MediSoft* program.

14. Make a backup copy of your data disk.

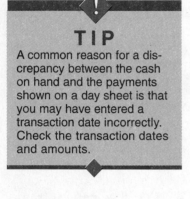

TIP

A common reason for a discrepancy between the cash on hand and the payments shown on a day sheet is that you may have entered a transaction date incorrectly. Check the transaction dates and amounts.

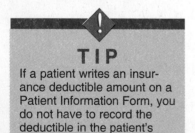

TIP

If a patient writes an insurance deductible amount on a Patient Information Form, you do not have to record the deductible in the patient's case record.

1. Remove Source Documents 27 through 38 on pages 211-234. Review the information provided on the source documents.

2. Start the *MediSoft* program.

3. Set the program date to **September 8, 1998** before entering the transactions from yesterday afternoon.

4. Record the following transactions from Tuesday using the information provided on Source Documents 27-30. Use the *Enter Transactions* option to record the procedure charges and payments. Print a walkout receipt for each patient.

   ♦ Enter the procedure charges and payment for Ethan Sampson (Source Document 27). Ethan is covered by his mother's (Caroline Sampson) insurance (Spalding Group Life and Health, Policy #: 36092, Group #: L409, Coverage: 80%). Remember to enter **09/08/98** for the transaction date and print a walkout receipt.

   ♦ Enter the information to record the transactions for Jo Black, who is a new patient (Source Documents 28 and 29).

   ♦ Record the procedure charges for Sarina Bell (Source Document 30). She is covered by her father's insurance policy. **Hint:** Look up the insurance policy information by reviewing one of Herbert Bell's case records.

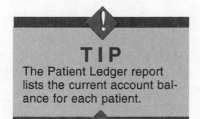

TIP
The Patient Ledger report lists the current account balance for each patient.

5. A patient, Hiro Tanaka, called the office to inquire about her account balance. Write the patient's account balance in the space provided. BALANCE: $_137.00_

6. Process the two checks received yesterday (Source Document 31).

7. Print a Patient Day Sheet and a Procedure Day Sheet for Tuesday, September 8, 1998.

✳8. Verify that you have entered the information correctly so that you can prepare a bank deposit slip. The cash on hand totals $572.50. If this amount does not match the information on the reports, find the error and make the necessary correction.

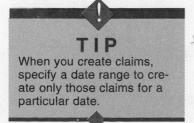

TIP
When you create claims, specify a date range to create only those claims for a particular date.

✳9. Create the insurance claim forms for the patient charges you just entered. Print the claims using the HCFA-1500 (Primary) form. Proof the claim forms you just printed.

10. Change the program date to **September 9, 1998** to enter today's transactions.

11. Process the transactions from this morning (Source Documents 32-38). Remember to print a walkout receipt for each patient.

    - Enter the procedure charge for John Gardiner (Source Document 32). His health insurance carrier is Ten County Health Cooperative (Policy #: 6397008, Group #: J10-32, Coverage: 100%).

    (will cont.) — - Record the new telephone number for Paul Ramos (Source Document 33).

    - Input the new patient information and enter the transactions for Sam Wu (Source Documents 34 and 35).

    - Enter the transactions for Paul Ramos who is a full-time student, not married, and currently not employed (Source Document 36). He is covered by his mother's health insurance. Maritza Ramos and her son are insured with Champus (Policy #: 15862283). Their insurance provides 100% coverage for approved procedure charges.

    - Record the procedure charge and payment for Ellen Barmenstein (Source Document 37). Be sure to enter a new case and apply the payment to this visit.

    - Record the procedure charge for Elizabeth Jones (Source Document 38). This visit is related to the previous case.

12. Exit the *MediSoft* program and make a backup copy of your data disk.

THURSDAY, SEPTEMBER 10, 1998 ◆

1. Remove and review Source Documents 39 through 46 on pages 235-250.

2. Start the *MediSoft* program.

3. Set the program date to **September 9, 1998** to enter the transactions from Wednesday afternoon.

4. Record the following transactions from Wednesday using the information provided on Source Documents 39-42. Print a walkout receipt for each patient.

    - Enter the procedure charges and payment for James Smith (Source Document 39).

    - Record the transactions for Joe Abate, a new patient (Source Documents 40 and 41).

◆ Record the procedure charge and payment for Sarabeth Smith (Source Document 42). Sarabeth, who is single, has her own insurance policy (Spalding Group Life and Health, Policy #: 03467, Group #: 2450, Coverage: 80%).

5. A patient, Herbert Bell, called the office to inquire about his account balance. Write the patient's account balance in the space provided. BALANCE: $30.00

6. Process the two checks received yesterday (Source Document 43).

✳ 7. Print a Patient Day Sheet and a Procedure Day Sheet for Wednesday, September 9, 1998.

✳ 8. Verify that you have entered the information correctly so that you can prepare a bank deposit slip. The cash and checks on hand should total $1,100.50. Make any necessary corrections.

9. Create and print the insurance claim forms for the patient charges.

10. Change the program date to **September 10, 1998** to enter today's transactions.

11. Process the transactions from this morning (Source Documents 44-46). Remember to print a walkout receipt for each patient.

◆ Enter the procedure charges for Maritza Ramos who has a Champus policy with 100% coverage (Source Document 44).

◆ Record the procedure charges and payment for Sarina Bell (Source Document 45). Apply the payment to this visit.

◆ Record the transactions for Jo Wong and apply the payment to this visit (Source Document 46).

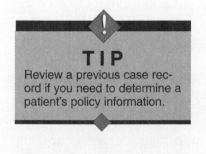

TIP

Review a previous case record if you need to determine a patient's policy information.

✳ 12. After reviewing the Patient Aging report and discussing the matter with the office manager, you decide to writeoff the amounts owed by Paula Ross and Winston Ward. **Hint:** Using the Transaction Entry screen, enter the patient's chart number and select an existing case. Choose to enter a new transaction. Enter the bad debt in the *Adjustment* folder using *05* for the adjustment code. Record the adjustment as a negative (-) amount in the *Amount* field and again when you apply the adjustment to charges. Make sure that the patient's balance is $0.00.

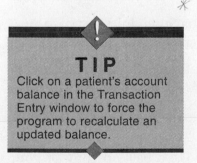

TIP

Click on a patient's account balance in the Transaction Entry window to force the program to recalculate an updated balance.

✳ 13. Print a separate Patient Ledger report for each of the patient's accounts you adjusted. Verify that their account balances are zero ($0.00).

14. Exit the *MediSoft* program and make a backup copy of your data disk.

1. Remove and review Source Documents 47 through 50 on pages 251-258.

2. Start the *MediSoft* program.

3. Set the program date to **September 10, 1998** to enter the transactions from Thursday afternoon.

4. Process the two checks received yesterday (Source Document 47).

5. Print a Patient Day Sheet and a Procedure Day Sheet for Thursday, September 10, 1998.

6. Verify that you have entered the information correctly so that you can prepare a bank deposit slip. The cash and checks on hand total $295.00. Make any necessary corrections.

7. Create and print the insurance claim forms for the patient charges.

8. Print patient statements for patients whose last names begin with G through L. Do **not** enter a date range filter when you print the statements.

9. Print a Patient Ledger report for all patients. Do not use a date range.

10. Print a Practice Analysis report. Use 09/04/98 through 09/10/98 for the report date range.

11. Change the program date to **September 11, 1998** to enter today's transactions.

12. Process the transactions from this morning (Source Documents 48-50). Remember to print a walkout receipt for each patient.

    ◆ Enter the procedure charges for Surendra Uzwahl, a new patient (Source Documents 48 and 49).

    ◆ Record the transactions for Jonathan Bell (Source Document 50). He is covered by his father's (Herbert Bell) U.S. Life and Health insurance (Policy #: 50632, Group #: 6209, Coverage: 80%).

13. Exit the *MediSoft* program and make a backup copy of your data disk.

14. Complete the Simulation Assessment Test if your instructor provided you with a copy of this test. Use the reports you printed this session to answer the questions on the test.

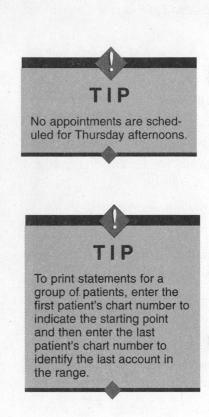

TIP

No appointments are scheduled for Thursday afternoons.

TIP

To print statements for a group of patients, enter the first patient's chart number to indicate the starting point and then enter the last patient's chart number to identify the last account in the range.

Source Documents

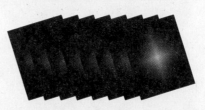

Use the source documents provided in this section to complete the tutorial (Source Documents 1-14, pages 159-186) and simulation (Source Documents 15-50, pages 187-258). Blank source documents are provided on pages 259-274 if you want to practice entering additional information.

Family Care Center
Patient Information Form

PERSONAL

Name (last, first): _Lomos, Juan_   Sex: ☑ Male
Address: _12 Briar Lane_   ☐ Female
Stephenson, OH 60089
Phone No.: _(614) 221-0202_   Marital Status: ☑ Married   ☐ Single
_(   )_   ☐ Separated ☐ Divorced
                                                   ☐ Widowed

Birth Date: _7/21/41_
Social Security No.: _716-83-0061_   Student Status: ☐ Full Time   ☑ Non-Student
                                                      ☐ Part Time

EMPLOYMENT

Employer: _Stephenson Wire Works_   Employed: ☑ Full Time
Address: _125 Stephenson Road_   ☐ Part Time
Stephenson, OH 60082   ☐ Not Employed
Phone No.: _(614) 525-0215_ Ext.: _____   ☐ Retired
                                                     Date: _____

INSURANCE

Primary
  Insurance Carrier: _Blue Cross/Blue Shield_   Co-Pay Amount: _____
Policy No.: _716830061_   Group No.: _126_   Percent Covered: _80_
Insured: _(same)_
Relationship
  to Insured: ☑ Self   ☐ Spouse   ☐ Child   ☐ Other
Secondary
  Insurance Carrier: _____   Co-Pay Amount: _____
Policy No.: _____   Group No.: _____   Percent Covered: _____
Insured: _____
Relationship
  to Insured: ☐ Self   ☐ Spouse   ☐ Child   ☐ Other

OTHER

Reason for Visit: _Auto accident—back injury_
Known Allergies: _none_
Did another physician refer you to our office? ☐ Yes ☑ No   If yes, who? _____
Condition Related to: ☑ Auto Accident   ☐ Employment Accident   ☐ Other Accident
Date Accident Occurred: _8/9/98_   State Where Accident Occurred: _OH_

For office use only:
Chart No.: _____   Assigned Provider: _1_   Billing Code: _A_
Signature on File: ☐ Yes ☑ No

FAMILY CARE CENTER
Dr. Katherine Yan

Date: 9/4/98

Patient: Juan Lomos

Physician's Notes:

Condition related to automobile accident in Ohio, August 9, 1998.

Was hospitalized from August 9, 1998 to August 15, 1998.

Patient was totally disabled from August 9, 1998 to August 20, 1998.

Patient remained partially disabled from August 21 to September 2, 1998.

Family Care Center
Patient Information Form

PERSONAL

Name (last, first): _Lomos, Cedera_

Address: _12 Briar Lane_

Stephenson, OH 60089

Phone No.: _(614) 221-0202_

_(   )_

Birth Date: _5/21/46_

Social Security No.: _717-87-0054_

Sex: ☐ Male ☑ Female

Marital Status: ☑ Married ☐ Single ☐ Separated ☐ Divorced ☐ Widowed

Student Status: ☐ Full Time ☑ Non-Student ☐ Part Time

EMPLOYMENT

Employer: _Stephenson Wire Works_

Address: _125 Stephenson Road_

Stephenson, OH 60082

Phone No.: _(614) 525-0215_ Ext.: _____

Employed: ☑ Full Time ☐ Part Time ☐ Not Employed ☐ Retired

Date: _____

INSURANCE

Primary

Insurance Carrier: _Blue Cross/Blue Shield_

Policy No.: _716830061_ Group No.: _126_

Insured: _Juan Lomos_

Relationship to Insured: ☐ Self ☑ Spouse ☐ Child ☐ Other

Co-Pay Amount: _____

Percent Covered: _80_

Secondary

Insurance Carrier: _Physician Alliance of Ohio_

Policy No.: _621382_ Group No.: _A435_

Insured: _Cedera Lomos_

Relationship to Insured: ☑ Self ☐ Spouse ☐ Child ☐ Other

Co-Pay Amount: _____

Percent Covered: _90_

OTHER

Reason for Visit: _persistent cough_

Known Allergies: _penicillin_

Did another physician refer you to our office? ☐ Yes ☑ No If yes, who? _____

Condition Related to: ☐ Auto Accident ☐ Employment Accident ☐ Other Accident

Date Accident Occurred: _____ State Where Accident Occurred: _____

For office use only:

Chart No.: _____ Assigned Provider: _1_ Billing Code: _A_

Signature on File: ☐ Yes ☑ No

Family Care Center
Patient Information Form

PERSONAL

Name (last, first): _Lomos, Lisa_

Address: _12 Briar Lane_

Stephenson, OH 60089

Phone No.: _(614) 221-0202_

_(   )_

Birth Date: _6/3/93_

Social Security No.: _212-55-3311_

Sex: ☐ Male
☑ Female

Marital Status:
☐ Married ☑ Single
☐ Separated ☐ Divorced
☐ Widowed

Student Status: ☐ Full Time ☑ Non-Student
☐ Part Time

EMPLOYMENT

Employer: _____

Address: _____

_____

Phone No.: (   )   Ext.: _____

Employed: ☐ Full Time
☐ Part Time
☑ Not Employed
☐ Retired

Date: _____

INSURANCE

Primary

Insurance Carrier: _Blue Cross/Blue Shield_

Policy No.: _716830061_   Group No.: _126_

Insured: _Juan Lomos_

Relationship to Insured: ☐ Self ☐ Spouse ☑ Child ☐ Other

Co-Pay Amount: _____

Percent Covered: _80_

Secondary

Insurance Carrier: _Physician Alliance of Ohio_

Policy No.: _621382_   Group No.: _A435_

Insured: _Cedera Lomos_

Relationship to Insured: ☐ Self ☐ Spouse ☑ Child ☐ Other

Co-Pay Amount: _____

Percent Covered: _90_

OTHER

Reason for Visit: _routine well-child checkup_

Known Allergies: _none_

Did another physician refer you to our office? ☐ Yes ☑ No   If yes, who? _____

Condition Related to: ☐ Auto Accident ☐ Employment Accident ☐ Other Accident

Date Accident Occurred: _____   State Where Accident Occurred: _____

For office use only:

Chart No.: _____   Assigned Provider: _1_   Billing Code: _A_

Signature on File: ☐ Yes ☑ No

Family Care Center
Patient Information Form

PERSONAL

Name (last, first): *Wong, Angela*

Address: *10 Maytime Lane, Apt. 3*

Stephenson, OH 60089

Phone No.: *(614) 212-0808*

( )

Birth Date: *3/8/78*

Social Security No.: *123-62-2111*

Sex:
- ❏ Male
- ☑ Female

Marital Status:
- ❏ Married   ☑ Single
- ❏ Separated   ❏ Divorced
- ❏ Widowed

Student Status:
- ☑ Full Time   ❏ Non-Student
- ❏ Part Time

EMPLOYMENT

Employer: _____

Address: _____

_____

Phone No.: ( ) _____ Ext.: _____

Employed:
- ❏ Full Time
- ❏ Part Time
- ☑ Not Employed
- ❏ Retired

Date: _____

INSURANCE

Primary

Insurance Carrier: *Champus (Medicare)*

Policy No.: *397214A*   Group No.: *126*

Insured: *Peter Wong   320 Fourth St. Stephenson, OH 60089*

Relationship
to Insured: ❏ Self   ❏ Spouse   ☑ Child   ❏ Other

Co-Pay Amount: _____

Percent Covered: _____

Secondary

Insurance Carrier: _____

Policy No.: _____ Group No.: _____

Insured: _____

Relationship
to Insured: ❏ Self   ❏ Spouse   ❏ Child   ❏ Other

Co-Pay Amount: _____

Percent Covered: _____

OTHER

Reason for Visit: *checkup*

Known Allergies: *none*

Did another physician refer you to our office?   ❏ Yes   ☑ No   If yes, who? _____

Condition Related to: ❏ Auto Accident   ❏ Employment Accident   ❏ Other Accident

Date Accident Occurred: _____   State Where Accident Occurred: _____

For office use only:

Chart No.: _____   Assigned Provider: *1*   Billing Code: *A*

Signature on File: ❏ Yes   ☑ No

FAMILY CARE CENTER
THINGS TO DO TODAY

Notes:

John Fitzwilliams changed jobs. His new employer is Jenny Designs.

Work phone: (614) 876-1421

FAMILY CARE CENTER

Dr. Katherine Yan

Date: _9/4/98_

Patient: _Herbert Mitchell_

Physician's Notes:

Patient was hospitalized for angina from August 8 through September 2, 1998.

Medicare representative was contacted and authorized treatment.

Authorization number: 128-33821

Outside lab work bill for $300.00.

Family Care Center
285 Stephenson Boulevard
Stephenson, OH 60089
(614) 555-0100

Provider: Dr. Katherine Yan   **ID #**: 84021   **S.S. #**: 810-99-1110

Patient: *Lomos, Cedera*   **Chart #**: *LOMCE000*   **Document**:

Address: **Phone**:   **Date**: *9/4/98*

CODE	DESCRIPTION	X
New Patient		
99201	OF—New Patient Focused	
99202	OF—New Patient Expanded	
99203	OF—New Patient, Complete Physical	
Established Patient		
99213	OF—Established Patient Expanded	
99214	OF—Established Patient Routine Exam	
99215	OF—Established Patient Complex	
99211	OF—Established Patient Minimal	
99212	OF—Established Patient Focused	
Procedures		
85007	Manual WBC	
85651	Erythrocyte Sed Rate—ESR	
86403	Strep Test, Rapid	
86585	Tine Test	
87072	Strep Culture	
87086	Urine Culture	
93000	Electroencephalogram—EEG	
93015	Treadmill Stress Test	
90782	Injection	
Other Procedures		
99204	*OF — New Patient Mod.*	✓

Payments:

Diagnosis/ICD-9: *Sinusitis—chronic*

Remarks: **Today's Charges**: $

Next Appointment: **Amount Paid**: $

Family Care Center
285 Stephenson Boulevard
Stephenson, OH 60089
(614) 555-0100

Provider: Dr. Katherine Yan	**ID #**: 84021	**S.S. #**: 810-99-1110

Patient: *Lomos, Lisa*	**Chart #**: *LOMLI000*	**Document**:
Address:	**Phone**:	**Date**: *9/4/98*

CODE	DESCRIPTION	X
New Patient		
99201	OF—New Patient Focused	
99202	OF—New Patient Expanded	
99203	OF—New Patient, Complete Physical	✓
Established Patient		
99213	OF—Established Patient Expanded	
99214	OF—Established Patient Routine Exam	
99215	OF—Established Patient Complex	
99211	OF—Established Patient Minimal	
99212	OF—Established Patient Focused	
Procedures		
85007	Manual WBC	
85651	Erythrocyte Sed Rate—ESR	
86403	Strep Test, Rapid	
86585	Tine Test	
87072	Strep Culture	
87086	Urine Culture	
93000	Electroencephalogram—EEG	
93015	Treadmill Stress Test	
90782	Injection	
Other Procedures		
	MMR	✓

Payments:

Diagnosis/ICD-9: *Normal state—patient fears unfounded Immunization*

Remarks:	**Today's Charges**:	$
Next Appointment:	**Amount Paid**:	$

Family Care Center
285 Stephenson Boulevard
Stephenson, OH 60089
(614) 555-0100

Provider: Dr. Katherine Yan   **ID #**: 84021   **S.S. #**: 810-99-1110

Patient: *Patterson, Leila*   **Chart #**: *PATLE000*   **Document**:

Address: **Phone**:   **Date**: *9/4/98*

CODE	DESCRIPTION	X
New Patient		
99201	OF—New Patient Focused	
99202	OF—New Patient Expanded	
99203	OF—New Patient, Complete Physical	
Established Patient		
99213	OF—Established Patient Expanded	
99214	OF—Established Patient Routine Exam	
99215	OF—Established Patient Complex	
99211	OF—Established Patient Minimal	
99212	OF—Established Patient Focused	✓
Procedures		
85007	Manual WBC	
85651	Erythrocyte Sed Rate—ESR	
86403	Strep Test, Rapid	
86585	Tine Test	
87072	Strep Culture	
87086	Urine Culture	
93000	Electroencephalogram—EEG	
93015	Treadmill Stress Test	
90782	Injection	
Other Procedures		
	Cholesterol test	✓

Payments:

Diagnosis/ICD-9: *Hypercholesteremia*

Remarks: **Today's Charges**: $

Next Appointment: **Amount Paid**: $

Family Care Center
285 Stephenson Boulevard
Stephenson, OH 60089
(614) 555-0100

Provider: Dr. Katherine Yan   **ID #**: 84021   **S.S. #**: 810-99-1110

Patient: *Barmenstein, Ellen*   **Chart #**: *BAREL000*   **Document**:

Address: **Phone**:   **Date**: *9/4/98*

CODE	DESCRIPTION	X
New Patient		
99201	OF—New Patient Focused	
99202	OF—New Patient Expanded	
99203	OF—New Patient, Complete Physical	
Established Patient		
99213	OF—Established Patient Expanded	
99214	OF—Established Patient Routine Exam	✓
99215	OF—Established Patient Complex	
99211	OF—Established Patient Minimal	
99212	OF—Established Patient Focused	
Procedures		
85007	Manual WBC	
85651	Erythrocyte Sed Rate—ESR	
86403	Strep Test, Rapid	
86585	Tine Test	
87072	Strep Culture	
87086	Urine Culture	
93000	Electroencephalogram—EEG	
93015	Treadmill Stress Test	
90782	Injection	
Other Procedures		

Payments:

Diagnosis/ICD-9: *Routine physical exam*

Remarks: **Today's Charges**: $

Next Appointment: **Amount Paid**: $

Family Care Center
285 Stephenson Boulevard
Stephenson, OH 60089
(614) 555-0100

Provider: Dr. Katherine Yan   **ID #:** 84021   **S.S. #:** 810-99-1110

Patient: *Smolowski, Jim*   **Chart #:** *SMOJJ000*   **Document:**

Address: **Phone:**   **Date:** *9/4/98*

CODE	DESCRIPTION	X
New Patient		
99201	OF—New Patient Focused	
99202	OF—New Patient Expanded	
99203	OF—New Patient, Complete Physical	
Established Patient		
99213	OF—Established Patient Expanded	
99214	OF—Established Patient Routine Exam	✓
99215	OF—Established Patient Complex	
99211	OF—Established Patient Minimal	
99212	OF—Established Patient Focused	
Procedures		
85007	Manual WBC	
85651	Erythrocyte Sed Rate—ESR	
86403	Strep Test, Rapid	
86585	Tine Test	
87072	Strep Culture	
87086	Urine Culture	
93000	Electroencephalogram—EEG	✓
93015	Treadmill Stress Test	
90782	Injection	
Other Procedures		
	Glucose—quantitative	✓

Payments: *Received $75, Check #345*

Diagnosis/ICD-9: *Hyperglycemia*

Remarks: **Today's Charges:** $ *170.00*

Next Appointment: **Amount Paid:** $ *75.00*

Family Care Center
285 Stephenson Boulevard
Stephenson, OH 60089
(614) 555-0100

Provider: Dr. Katherine Yan **ID #**: 84021 **S.S. #**: 810-99-1110

Patient: *Wong, Li Yu* **Chart #:** *WONLI000* **Document:**

Address: **Phone:** **Date:** *9/4/98*

CODE	DESCRIPTION	X
New Patient		
99201	OF—New Patient Focused	
99202	OF—New Patient Expanded	
99203	OF—New Patient, Complete Physical	
Established Patient		
99213	OF—Established Patient Expanded	
99214	OF—Established Patient Routine Exam	
99215	OF—Established Patient Complex	
99211	OF—Established Patient Minimal	✓
99212	OF—Established Patient Focused	
Procedures		
85007	Manual WBC	
85651	Erythrocyte Sed Rate—ESR	
86403	Strep Test, Rapid	
86585	Tine Test	
87072	Strep Culture	
87086	Urine Culture	
93000	Electroencephalogram—EEG	
93015	Treadmill Stress Test	
90782	Injection	
Other Procedures		

Payments: *Received $10, Cash*

Diagnosis/ICD-9: *Bursitis (shoulder)*

Remarks: **Today's Charges:** *$ 50.00*

Next Appointment: **Amount Paid:** *$ 10.00*

Family Care Center
285 Stephenson Boulevard
Stephenson, OH 60089
(614) 555-0100

Provider: Dr. Katherine Yan   **ID #:** 84021   **S.S. #:** 810-99-1110

Patient: *Wong, Jo*   **Chart #:** *WONJO000*   **Document:**

Address: **Phone:**   **Date:** *9/4/98*

CODE	DESCRIPTION	X
New Patient		
99201	OF—New Patient Focused	
99202	OF—New Patient Expanded	
99203	OF—New Patient, Complete Physical	
Established Patient		
99213	OF—Established Patient Expanded	
99214	OF—Established Patient Routine Exam	
99215	OF—Established Patient Complex	
99211	OF—Established Patient Minimal	
99212	OF—Established Patient Focused	✓
Procedures		
85007	Manual WBC	
85651	Erythrocyte Sed Rate—ESR	
86403	Strep Test, Rapid	
86585	Tine Test	
87072	Strep Culture	
87086	Urine Culture	
93000	Electroencephalogram—EEG	
93015	Treadmill Stress Test	
90782	Injection	
Other Procedures		
	CBC with Diff	✓

Payments: *Received $20, Cash*

Diagnosis/ICD-9: *Upper respiratory infection—bronchitis*

Remarks: **Today's Charges:** $ *70.00*

Next Appointment: **Amount Paid:** $ *20.00*

Family Care Center
285 Stephenson Boulevard
Stephenson, OH 60089
(614) 555-0100

Provider: Dr. Katherine Yan	**ID #**: 84021	**S.S. #**: 810-99-1110

Patient: Bell, Janine	**Chart #:** BELJA000	**Document:**
Address:	**Phone:**	**Date:** 9/4/98

CODE	DESCRIPTION	X
New Patient		
99201	OF—New Patient Focused	
99202	OF—New Patient Expanded	
99203	OF—New Patient, Complete Physical	
Established Patient		
99213	OF—Established Patient Expanded	
99214	OF—Established Patient Routine Exam	
99215	OF—Established Patient Complex	
99211	OF—Established Patient Minimal	✓
99212	OF—Established Patient Focused	
Procedures		
85007	Manual WBC	
85651	Erythrocyte Sed Rate—ESR	
86403	Strep Test, Rapid	
86585	Tine Test	
87072	Strep Culture	
87086	Urine Culture	
93000	Electroencephalogram—EEG	
93015	Treadmill Stress Test	
90782	Injection	
Other Procedures		

Payments: Received $50, Check #33

Diagnosis/ICD-9: Diabetes Mellitus

Remarks:

Next Appointment: September 24, 1998

Today's Charges: $ 50.00

Amount Paid: $ 50.00

Family Care Center
285 Stephenson Boulevard
Stephenson, OH 60089
(614) 555-0100

Provider: Dr. Katherine Yan   **ID #:** 84021   **S.S. #:** 810-99-1110

Patient: *Suarez, Felix*   **Chart #:** *SUAFE000*   **Document:**

Address: **Phone:**   **Date:** *9/4/98*

CODE	DESCRIPTION	X
New Patient		
99201	OF—New Patient Focused	
99202	OF—New Patient Expanded	
99203	OF—New Patient, Complete Physical	
Established Patient		
99213	OF—Established Patient Expanded	
99214	OF—Established Patient Routine Exam	
99215	OF—Established Patient Complex	
99211	OF—Established Patient Minimal	
99212	OF—Established Patient Focused	✓
Procedures		
85007	Manual WBC	
85651	Erythrocyte Sed Rate—ESR	
86403	Strep Test, Rapid	
86585	Tine Test	
87072	Strep Culture	
87086	Urine Culture	
93000	Electroencephalogram—EEG	
93015	Treadmill Stress Test	
90782	Injection	
Other Procedures		

Payments:

Diagnosis/ICD-9: *Hemorrhoids*

Remarks: **Today's Charges:** $ *60.00*

Next Appointment: **Amount Paid:** $

Family Care Center
285 Stephenson Boulevard
Stephenson, OH 60089
(614) 555-0100

Provider: Dr. Katherine Yan   **ID #**: 84021   **S.S. #**: 810-99-1110

Patient: *Fitzwilliams, Sarah*   **Chart #**: *FITSA000*   **Document**:
Address: **Phone**:   **Date**: *9/4/98*

CODE	DESCRIPTION	X
New Patient		
99201	OF—New Patient Focused	
99202	OF—New Patient Expanded	
99203	OF—New Patient, Complete Physical	
Established Patient		
99213	OF—Established Patient Expanded	
99214	OF—Established Patient Routine Exam	
99215	OF—Established Patient Complex	
99211	OF—Established Patient Minimal	✓
99212	OF—Established Patient Focused	
Procedures		
85007	Manual WBC	
85651	Erythrocyte Sed Rate—ESR	
86403	Strep Test, Rapid	
86585	Tine Test	
87072	Strep Culture	
87086	Urine Culture	
93000	Electroencephalogram—EEG	
93015	Treadmill Stress Test	
90782	Injection	
Other Procedures		
	HDL Cholesterol	✓

Payments: *Received $75, Check #188*

Diagnosis/ICD-9: *Essential hypertension*

Remarks: **Today's Charges**: $ *75.00*

Next Appointment: **Amount Paid**: $ *75.00*

Family Care Center
285 Stephenson Boulevard
Stephenson, OH 60089
(614) 555-0100

Provider: Dr. Katherine Yan   **ID #:** 84021   **S.S. #:** 810-99-1110

Patient: *Johnson, Marion*   **Chart #:** *JOHMA000*   **Document:**

Address: **Phone:**   **Date:** *9/4/98*

CODE	DESCRIPTION	X
New Patient		
99201	OF—New Patient Focused	
99202	OF—New Patient Expanded	
99203	OF—New Patient, Complete Physical	
Established Patient		
99213	OF—Established Patient Expanded	
99214	OF—Established Patient Routine Exam	
99215	OF—Established Patient Complex	
99211	OF—Established Patient Minimal	
99212	OF—Established Patient Focused	✓
Procedures		
85007	Manual WBC	
85651	Erythrocyte Sed Rate—ESR	
86403	Strep Test, Rapid	
86585	Tine Test	
87072	Strep Culture	
87086	Urine Culture	
93000	Electroencephalogram—EEG	
93015	Treadmill Stress Test	
90782	Injection	
Other Procedures		
71020	*Chest X ray*	✓

Payments: *Received $120, Check #531*

Diagnosis/ICD-9: *Bronchitis, unqualified*

Remarks: **Today's Charges:** $ *120.00*

Next Appointment: **Amount Paid:** $ *120.00*

FAMILY CARE CENTER
THINGS TO DO TODAY

Notes:

Checks received on Friday, September 4, 1998:

From Rachel Brown for visit on August 22; Check #356, $55

From Herbert Bell's insurance carrier for visit on August 28; Check #10222, $120

From Felix Suarez's insurance carrier for visit on August 13; Check #8889, $88

From Herbert Mitchell's insurance carrier for visit on August 25; Check #10-227, $95

Family Care Center
Patient Information Form

PERSONAL

Name (last, first): _Andrews, Darla_

Address: _1 West 8th Street_

Stephenson, OH 60089

Phone No.: _(614)241-3321_

_( )_

Birth Date: _6/8/67_

Social Security No.: _332-49-0432_

Sex: ☐ Male ☑ Female

Marital Status: ☑ Married ☐ Single ☐ Separated ☐ Divorced ☐ Widowed

Student Status: ☐ Full Time ☑ Non-Student ☐ Part Time

EMPLOYMENT

Employer: _Wymark Drugs_

Address: _100 Main Street_

Stephenson, OH 60087

Phone No.: _(614)221-7893_ Ext.: _____

Employed: ☑ Full Time ☐ Part Time ☐ Not Employed ☐ Retired

Date: _____

INSURANCE

Primary

Insurance Carrier: _Spalding Group Life_

Policy No.: _8831_ Group No.: _203_

Insured: _Bill Andrews (same address)_

Co-Pay Amount: _____

Percent Covered: _80_

$200 deductible

Relationship to Insured: ☐ Self ☑ Spouse ☐ Child ☐ Other

Secondary

Insurance Carrier: _Ohio Central Health_

Policy No.: _1122191_ Group No.: _83_

Insured: _Darla Andrews_

Co-Pay Amount: _____

Percent Covered: _____

Relationship to Insured: ☑ Self ☐ Spouse ☐ Child ☐ Other

OTHER

Reason for Visit: _Chest pain_

Known Allergies: _none_

Did another physician refer you to our office? ☐ Yes ☑ No If yes, who? _____

Condition Related to: ☐ Auto Accident ☐ Employment Accident ☐ Other Accident

Date Accident Occurred: _____ State Where Accident Occurred: _____

For office use only:

Chart No.: _____ Assigned Provider: _1_ Billing Code: _A_

Signature on File: ☐ Yes ☑ No

Family Care Center
Patient Information Form

PERSONAL

Name (last, first): _Andrews, Bill_

Sex: ☑ Male ☐ Female

Address: _1 West 8th Street_

Stephenson, OH 60089

Phone No.: _(614) 221-3321_

_(   )_

Marital Status: ☑ Married ☐ Single ☐ Separated ☐ Divorced ☐ Widowed

Birth Date: _12/1/64_

Social Security No.: _341-59-9392_

Student Status: ☐ Full Time ☐ Part Time ☑ Non-Student

EMPLOYMENT

Employer: _East Tire Company_

Address: _Route 8_

Stephenson, OH 60087

Phone No.: _(614) 922-2984_ Ext.: _____

Employed: ☑ Full Time ☐ Part Time ☐ Not Employed ☐ Retired

Date: _____

INSURANCE

Primary

Insurance Carrier: _Spalding Group Life_

Policy No.: _8831_ Group No.: _203_

Insured: _Bill Andrews_

Co-Pay Amount: _____

Percent Covered: _80_

$200 deductible

Relationship to Insured: ☑ Self ☐ Spouse ☐ Child ☐ Other

Secondary

Insurance Carrier: _____

Policy No.: _____ Group No.: _____

Insured: _____

Co-Pay Amount: _____

Percent Covered: _____

Relationship to Insured: ☐ Self ☐ Spouse ☐ Child ☐ Other

OTHER

Reason for Visit: _Routine physical_

Known Allergies: _penicillin_

Did another physician refer you to our office? ☐ Yes ☑ No If yes, who? _____

Condition Related to: ☐ Auto Accident ☐ Employment Accident ☐ Other Accident

Date Accident Occurred: _____ State Where Accident Occurred: _____

For office use only:

Chart No.: _____ Assigned Provider: _1_ Billing Code: _A_

Signature on File: ☐ Yes ☑ No

FAMILY CARE CENTER
THINGS TO DO TODAY

Notes:

James Smith has a new address:

100 Meadowlark Lane

Stephenson, OH 60089

Family Care Center
285 Stephenson Boulevard
Stephenson, OH 60089
(614) 555-0100

Provider: Dr. Katherine Yan   **ID #**: 84021   **S.S. #**: 810-99-1110

Patient: *Andrews, Darla*   **Chart #**: *ANDDA000*   **Document**:

Address: **Phone**:   **Date**: *9/8/98*

CODE	DESCRIPTION	X
New Patient		
99201	OF—New Patient Focused	
99202	OF—New Patient Expanded	
99203	OF—New Patient, Complete Physical	
Established Patient		
99213	OF—Established Patient Expanded	
99214	OF—Established Patient Routine Exam	
99215	OF—Established Patient Complex	
99211	OF—Established Patient Minimal	
99212	OF—Established Patient Focused	✓
Procedures		
85007	Manual WBC	
85651	Erythrocyte Sed Rate—ESR	
86403	Strep Test, Rapid	
86585	Tine Test	
87072	Strep Culture	
87086	Urine Culture	
93000	Electroencephalogram—EEG	
93015	Treadmill Stress Test	
90782	Injection	
Other Procedures		
71020	*Chest X ray*	✓

Payments: *Received $24, Check #123*

Diagnosis/ICD-9: *Bronchopneumonia*

Remarks: **Today's Charges**: $ *120.00*

Next Appointment: **Amount Paid**: $ *24.00*

Family Care Center
285 Stephenson Boulevard
Stephenson, OH 60089
(614) 555-0100

Provider: Dr. Katherine Yan   **ID #**: 84021   **S.S. #**: 810-99-1110

Patient: *Andrews, Bill*   **Chart #**: *ANDBI000*   **Document**:

Address: **Phone**:   **Date**: *9/8/98*

CODE	DESCRIPTION	X
New Patient		
99201	OF—New Patient Focused	
99202	OF—New Patient Expanded	
99203	OF—New Patient, Complete Physical	
Established Patient		
99213	OF—Established Patient Expanded	
99214	OF—Established Patient Routine Exam	✓
99215	OF—Established Patient Complex	
99211	OF—Established Patient Minimal	
99212	OF—Established Patient Focused	
Procedures		
85007	Manual WBC	
85651	Erythrocyte Sed Rate—ESR	
86403	Strep Test, Rapid	
86585	Tine Test	
87072	Strep Culture	
87086	Urine Culture	
93000	Electroencephalogram—EEG	
93015	Treadmill Stress Test	
90782	Injection	
Other Procedures		

Payments: *Received $16, Check #124*

Diagnosis/ICD-9: *Physical exam*

Remarks: **Today's Charges**: $ *80.00*

Next Appointment: **Amount Paid**: $ *16.00*

Family Care Center
285 Stephenson Boulevard
Stephenson, OH 60089
(614) 555-0100

Provider: Dr. Katherine Yan **ID #**: 84021 **S.S. #**: 810-99-1110

Patient: *Lomos, Cedera* **Chart #**: *LOMCE000* **Document**:
Address: **Phone**: **Date**: *9/8/98*

CODE	DESCRIPTION	X
New Patient		
99201	OF—New Patient Focused	
99202	OF—New Patient Expanded	
99203	OF—New Patient, Complete Physical	
Established Patient		
99213	OF—Established Patient Expanded	
99214	OF—Established Patient Routine Exam	
99215	OF—Established Patient Complex	
99211	OF—Established Patient Minimal	✓
99212	OF—Established Patient Focused	
Procedures		
85007	Manual WBC	
85651	Erythrocyte Sed Rate—ESR	
86403	Strep Test, Rapid	
86585	Tine Test	
87072	Strep Culture	
87086	Urine Culture	
93000	Electroencephalogram—EEG	
93015	Treadmill Stress Test	
90782	Injection	
Other Procedures		

Payments: *Received $50, Check #1204*

Diagnosis/ICD-9: *Acute sinusitis*

Remarks: **Today's Charges**: $ *50.00*

Next Appointment: **Amount Paid**: $ *50.00*

Family Care Center
285 Stephenson Boulevard
Stephenson, OH 60089
(614) 555-0100

Provider: Dr. Katherine Yan   **ID #**: 84021   **S.S. #**: 810-99-1110

Patient: *Feldman, Stanley*   **Chart #**: *FELST000*   **Document**:

Address: **Phone**:   **Date**: *9/8/98*

CODE	DESCRIPTION	X
New Patient		
99201	OF—New Patient Focused	
99202	OF—New Patient Expanded	
99203	OF—New Patient, Complete Physical	
Established Patient		
99213	OF—Established Patient Expanded	
99214	OF—Established Patient Routine Exam	
99215	OF—Established Patient Complex	
99211	OF—Established Patient Minimal	
99212	OF—Established Patient Focused	
Procedures		
85007	Manual WBC	
85651	Erythrocyte Sed Rate—ESR	
86403	Strep Test, Rapid	
86585	Tine Test	
87072	Strep Culture	
87086	Urine Culture	
93000	Electroencephalogram—EEG	
93015	Treadmill Stress Test	
90782	Injection	
Other Procedures		
80061		✓

Payments: *Received $20, Check #991*

Diagnosis/ICD-9: *Hypercholesteremia*

Remarks: **Today's Charges**: $ *20.00*

Next Appointment: **Amount Paid**: $ *20.00*

Family Care Center
285 Stephenson Boulevard
Stephenson, OH 60089
(614) 555-0100

Provider: Dr. Katherine Yan   **ID #:** 84021   **S.S. #:** 810-99-1110

Patient: *Sampson, Ethan*   **Chart #:** *SAME1000*   **Document:**

Address: **Phone:**   **Date:** *9/8/98*

CODE	DESCRIPTION	X
New Patient		
99201	OF—New Patient Focused	
99202	OF—New Patient Expanded	
99203	OF—New Patient, Complete Physical	
Established Patient		
99213	OF—Established Patient Expanded	
99214	OF—Established Patient Routine Exam	✓
99215	OF—Established Patient Complex	
99211	OF—Established Patient Minimal	
99212	OF—Established Patient Focused	
Procedures		
85007	Manual WBC	
85651	Erythrocyte Sed Rate—ESR	
86403	Strep Test, Rapid	
86585	Tine Test	
87072	Strep Culture	
87086	Urine Culture	
93000	Electroencephalogram—EEG	
93015	Treadmill Stress Test	
90782	Injection	
Other Procedures		
73090	*Forearm X ray AP & Lat*	✓

Payments: *Received $130, Check #129*

Diagnosis/ICD-9: *Sprain — No cast*

Remarks: **Today's Charges:** *$130.00*

Next Appointment: **Amount Paid:** *$130.00*

Family Care Center
Patient Information Form

PERSONAL

Name (last, first): _Black, Jo_

Address: _3 Parkway Road_

Stephenson, OH 60089

Phone No.: _(614) 555-8989_

_( )_

Birth Date: _1/11/47_

Social Security No.: _321-22-8787_

Sex: ☐ Male
☑ Female

Marital Status: ☐ Married ☑ Single
☐ Separated ☐ Divorced
☐ Widowed

Student Status: ☐ Full Time ☑ Non-Student
☐ Part Time

EMPLOYMENT

Employer: _Dr. Walter Weis_

Address: _Stephenson General Hospital_

Stephenson, OH 60086

Phone No.: _(614) 555-0101_   Ext.: _____

Employed: ☑ Full Time
☐ Part Time
☐ Not Employed
☐ Retired

Date: _____

INSURANCE

Primary

Insurance Carrier: _Blue Cross/Blue Shield_

Policy No.: _321228787_   Group No.: _____

Insured: _Jo Black,_

Relationship
to Insured: ☑ Self ☐ Spouse ☐ Child ☐ Other

Co-Pay Amount: _____

Percent Covered: _80_

$200 deductible

Secondary

Insurance Carrier: _____

Policy No.: _____   Group No.: _____

Insured: _____

Relationship
to Insured: ☐ Self ☐ Spouse ☐ Child ☐ Other

Co-Pay Amount: _____

Percent Covered: _____

OTHER

Reason for Visit: _____

Known Allergies: _____

Did another physician refer you to our office? ☑ Yes ☐ No   If yes, who? _Dr. Walter Weis_

Condition Related to: ☐ Auto Accident   ☐ Employment Accident   ☐ Other Accident

Date Accident Occurred: _____   State Where Accident Occurred: _____

For office use only:

Chart No.: _____   Assigned Provider: _1_   Billing Code: _A_

Signature on File: ☐ Yes ☑ No

Family Care Center
285 Stephenson Boulevard
Stephenson, OH 60089
(614) 555-0100

Provider: Dr. Katherine Yan	**ID #**: 84021	**S.S. #**: 810-99-1110

Patient: *Black, Jo*	**Chart #**: *BLAJO000*	**Document**:
Address:	**Phone**:	**Date**: *9/8/98*

CODE	DESCRIPTION	X
New Patient		
99201	OF—New Patient Focused	
99202	OF—New Patient Expanded	
99203	OF—New Patient, Complete Physical	✓
Established Patient		
99213	OF—Established Patient Expanded	
99214	OF—Established Patient Routine Exam	
99215	OF—Established Patient Complex	
99211	OF—Established Patient Minimal	
99212	OF—Established Patient Focused	
Procedures		
85007	Manual WBC	
85651	Erythrocyte Sed Rate—ESR	
86403	Strep Test, Rapid	
86585	Tine Test	
87072	Strep Culture	
87086	Urine Culture	
93000	Electroencephalogram—EEG	
93015	Treadmill Stress Test	
90782	Injection	
Other Procedures		

Payments: *Received $200, Check #566*

Diagnosis/ICD-9: *Arrhythmia*

Remarks:	**Today's Charges**:	$ *200.00*
Next Appointment:	**Amount Paid**:	$ *200.00*

Family Care Center
285 Stephenson Boulevard
Stephenson, OH 60089
(614) 555-0100

Provider: Dr. Katherine Yan   **ID #**: 84021   **S.S. #**: 810-99-1110

Patient: *Bell, Sarina*   **Chart #**: *BELSA001*   **Document**:

Address: **Phone**:   **Date**: *9/8/98*

CODE	DESCRIPTION	X
New Patient		
99201	OF—New Patient Focused	
99202	OF—New Patient Expanded	
99203	OF—New Patient, Complete Physical	
Established Patient		
99213	OF—Established Patient Expanded	
99214	OF—Established Patient Routine Exam	
99215	OF—Established Patient Complex	
99211	OF—Established Patient Minimal	✓
99212	OF—Established Patient Focused	
Procedures		
85007	Manual WBC	
85651	Erythrocyte Sed Rate—ESR	
86403	Strep Test, Rapid	✓
86585	Tine Test	
87072	Strep Culture	
87086	Urine Culture	
93000	Electroencephalogram—EEG	
93015	Treadmill Stress Test	
90782	Injection	
Other Procedures		

Payments:

Diagnosis/ICD-9: *Strep, sore throat*

Remarks: **Today's Charges**: $ *65.00*

Next Appointment: **Amount Paid**: $

FAMILY CARE CENTER
THINGS TO DO TODAY

Notes:

Checks received on Tuesday, September 8, 1998:

From Caroline Sampson for visit on August 6; Check #1002, $27.50

From Li Yu Wong for visits on August 20 and September 4; Check #189, $105.00

Family Care Center
285 Stephenson Boulevard
Stephenson, OH 60089
(614) 555-0100

Provider: Dr. Katherine Yan   **ID #:** 84021   **S.S. #:** 810-99-1110

Patient: *Gardiner, John*   **Chart #:** *GARJO000*   **Document:**

Address: **Phone:**   **Date:** *9/9/98*

CODE	DESCRIPTION	X
New Patient		
99201	OF—New Patient Focused	
99202	OF—New Patient Expanded	
99203	OF—New Patient, Complete Physical	
Established Patient		
99213	OF—Established Patient Expanded	
99214	OF—Established Patient Routine Exam	
99215	OF—Established Patient Complex	
99211	OF—Established Patient Minimal	✓
99212	OF—Established Patient Focused	
Procedures		
85007	Manual WBC	
85651	Erythrocyte Sed Rate—ESR	
86403	Strep Test, Rapid	
86585	Tine Test	
87072	Strep Culture	
87086	Urine Culture	
93000	Electroencephalogram—EEG	
93015	Treadmill Stress Test	
90782	Injection	
Other Procedures		

Payments:

Diagnosis/ICD-9: *Flu*

Remarks: **Today's Charges:** $ *50.00*

Next Appointment: **Amount Paid:** $

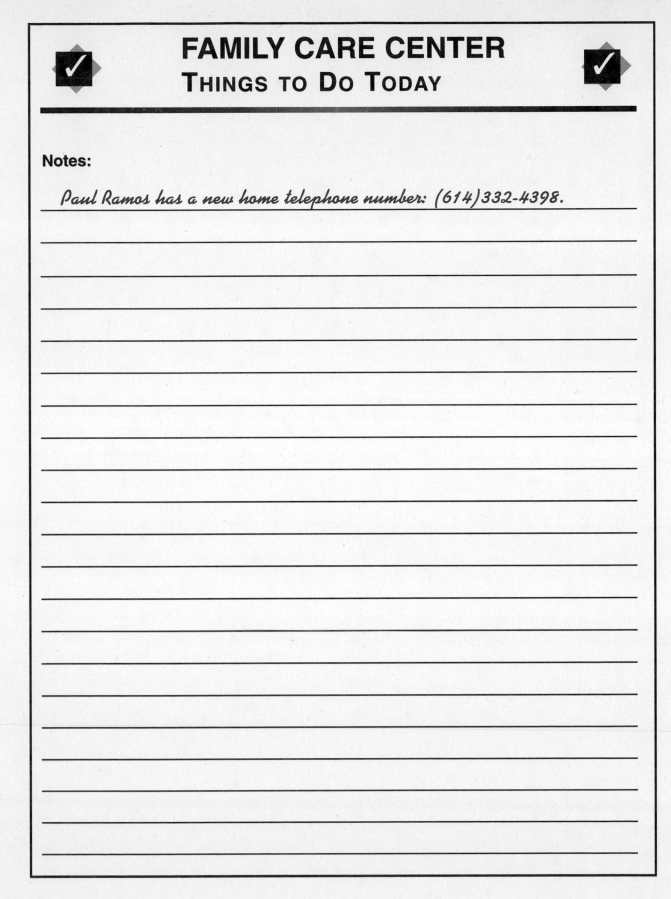

✓ **FAMILY CARE CENTER**
THINGS TO DO TODAY

Notes:

Paul Ramos has a new home telephone number: (614)332-4398.

Family Care Center
Patient Information Form

PERSONAL

Name (last, first): _Wu, Sam_   Sex: ☑ Male

Address: _4701 Plymouth Avenue_   ☐ Female

Stephenson, OH 60089

Phone No.: _(614)931-3319_   Marital Status: ☐ Married   ☐ Single

_(   )_   ☑ Separated   ☐ Divorced

                                                        ☐ Widowed

Birth Date: _8/8/41_

Social Security No.: _381-77-9138_   Student Status: ☐ Full Time   ☑ Non-Student

                                                              ☐ Part Time

EMPLOYMENT

                                                        Employed: ☑ Full Time

Employer: _Western Telephone_   ☐ Part Time

Address: _126 Grand Army Circle_   ☐ Not Employed

Stephenson, OH 60082   ☐ Retired

Phone No.: _(614)555-8811_   Ext.: _____   Date: _____

INSURANCE

Primary
Insurance Carrier: _U.S. Life & Health_   Co-Pay Amount: _____

Policy No.: _381779183_   Group No.: _931_   Percent Covered: _80_

Insured: _____

Relationship
to Insured: ☑ Self   ☐ Spouse   ☐ Child   ☐ Other

Secondary
Insurance Carrier: _____   Co-Pay Amount: _____

Policy No.: _____   Group No.: _____   Percent Covered: _____

Insured: _____

Relationship
to Insured: ☐ Self   ☐ Spouse   ☐ Child   ☐ Other

OTHER

Reason for Visit: _Arm hurts when moved_

Known Allergies: _____

Did another physician refer you to our office?   ☑ Yes   ☐ No   If yes, who? _Dr. Gearhart_

Condition Related to: ☑ Auto Accident   ☐ Employment Accident   ☐ Other Accident

Date Accident Occurred: _9/7/98_   State Where Accident Occurred: _OH_

For office use only:

Chart No.: _____   Assigned Provider: _1_   Billing Code: _A_

Signature on File: ☐ Yes   ☑ No

Family Care Center
285 Stephenson Boulevard
Stephenson, OH 60089
(614) 555-0100

Provider: Dr. Katherine Yan   **ID #**: 84021   **S.S. #**: 810-99-1110

Patient: Wu, Sam   **Chart #**: WUSA0000   **Document**:

Address: **Phone**:   **Date**: 9/9/98

CODE	DESCRIPTION	X
New Patient		
99201	OF—New Patient Focused	✓
99202	OF—New Patient Expanded	
99203	OF—New Patient, Complete Physical	
Established Patient		
99213	OF—Established Patient Expanded	
99214	OF—Established Patient Routine Exam	
99215	OF—Established Patient Complex	
99211	OF—Established Patient Minimal	
99212	OF—Established Patient Focused	
Procedures		
85007	Manual WBC	
85651	Erythrocyte Sed Rate—ESR	
86403	Strep Test, Rapid	
86585	Tine Test	
87072	Strep Culture	
87086	Urine Culture	
93000	Electroencephalogram—EEG	
93015	Treadmill Stress Test	
90782	Injection	
Other Procedures		
73070	Elbow X ray	✓
73090	Forearm X ray	✓

Payments: Received $240, Check #561

Diagnosis/ICD-9: Sprain — no cast

Remarks:

Next Appointment:

Today's Charges: $ 240.00

Amount Paid: $ 240.00

Family Care Center
285 Stephenson Boulevard
Stephenson, OH 60089
(614) 555-0100

Provider: Dr. Katherine Yan   **ID #**: 84021   **S.S. #**: 810-99-1110

Patient: *Ramos, Paul*   **Chart #**: *RAMPA000*   **Document**:

Address: **Phone**:   **Date**: *9/9/98*

CODE	DESCRIPTION	X
New Patient		
99201	OF—New Patient Focused	
99202	OF—New Patient Expanded	
99203	OF—New Patient, Complete Physical	
Established Patient		
99213	OF—Established Patient Expanded	
99214	OF—Established Patient Routine Exam	✓
99215	OF—Established Patient Complex	
99211	OF—Established Patient Minimal	
99212	OF—Established Patient Focused	
Procedures		
85007	Manual WBC	
85651	Erythrocyte Sed Rate—ESR	
86403	Strep Test, Rapid	
86585	Tine Test	
87072	Strep Culture	
87086	Urine Culture	
93000	Electroencephalogram—EEG	
93015	Treadmill Stress Test	
90782	Injection	
Other Procedures		
87076		✓

Payments: *Received $80, Cash*

Diagnosis/ICD-9: *Urinary tract infection*

Remarks: **Today's Charges**: $ *95.00*

Next Appointment: **Amount Paid**: $ *80.00*

Family Care Center
285 Stephenson Boulevard
Stephenson, OH 60089
(614) 555-0100

Provider: Dr. Katherine Yan   **ID #**: 84021   **S.S. #**: 810-99-1110

Patient: *Barmenstein, Ellen*   **Chart #**: *BAREL000*   **Document**:

Address: **Phone**:   **Date**: *9/9/98*

CODE	DESCRIPTION	X
New Patient		
99201	OF—New Patient Focused	
99202	OF—New Patient Expanded	
99203	OF—New Patient, Complete Physical	
Established Patient		
99213	OF—Established Patient Expanded	
99214	OF—Established Patient Routine Exam	
99215	OF—Established Patient Complex	
99211	OF—Established Patient Minimal	
99212	OF—Established Patient Focused	
Procedures		
85007	Manual WBC	
85651	Erythrocyte Sed Rate—ESR	
86403	Strep Test, Rapid	
86585	Tine Test	
87072	Strep Culture	
87086	Urine Culture	
93000	Electroencephalogram—EEG	
93015	Treadmill Stress Test	
90782	Injection	
Other Procedures		
90724		✓

Payments: *Received $12, Cash*

Diagnosis/ICD-9: *Immunization*

Remarks: **Today's Charges**: $ *12.00*

Next Appointment: **Amount Paid**: $ *12.00*

Family Care Center
285 Stephenson Boulevard
Stephenson, OH 60089
(614) 555-0100

Provider: Dr. Katherine Yan   **ID #:** 84021   **S.S. #:** 810-99-1110

Patient: *Jones, Elizabeth*   **Chart #:** *JONEL000*   **Document:**

Address: **Phone:**   **Date:** *9/9/98*

CODE	DESCRIPTION	X
New Patient		
99201	OF—New Patient Focused	
99202	OF—New Patient Expanded	
99203	OF—New Patient, Complete Physical	
Established Patient		
99213	OF—Established Patient Expanded	
99214	OF—Established Patient Routine Exam	
99215	OF—Established Patient Complex	
99211	OF—Established Patient Minimal	
99212	OF—Established Patient Focused	✓
Procedures		
85007	Manual WBC	
85651	Erythrocyte Sed Rate—ESR	
86403	Strep Test, Rapid	
86585	Tine Test	
87072	Strep Culture	
87086	Urine Culture	
93000	Electroencephalogram—EEG	
93015	Treadmill Stress Test	
90782	Injection	
Other Procedures		

Payments:

Diagnosis/ICD-9: *Laceration*

Remarks: **Today's Charges:** $ *60.00*

Next Appointment: **Amount Paid:** $

Family Care Center
285 Stephenson Boulevard
Stephenson, OH 60089
(614) 555-0100

Provider: Dr. Katherine Yan   **ID #:** 84021   **S.S. #:** 810-99-1110

Patient: *Smith, James L.*   **Chart #:** *SMIJA000*   **Document:**

Address: **Phone:**   **Date:** *9/9/98*

CODE	DESCRIPTION	X
New Patient		
99201	OF—New Patient Focused	
99202	OF—New Patient Expanded	
99203	OF—New Patient, Complete Physical	
Established Patient		
99213	OF—Established Patient Expanded	
99214	OF—Established Patient Routine Exam	
99215	OF—Established Patient Complex	✓
99211	OF—Established Patient Minimal	
99212	OF—Established Patient Focused	
Procedures		
85007	Manual WBC	
85651	Erythrocyte Sed Rate—ESR	
86403	Strep Test, Rapid	
86585	Tine Test	
87072	Strep Culture	
87086	Urine Culture	
93000	Electroencephalogram—EEG	
93015	Treadmill Stress Test	✓
90782	Injection	
Other Procedures		

Payments: *Received $100, Check #224*

Diagnosis/ICD-9: *Pain – chest*

Remarks: **Today's Charges:** $ *250.00*

Next Appointment: **Amount Paid:** $ *100.00*

Family Care Center
Patient Information Form

PERSONAL

Name (last, first): _Abate, Joe_

Address: _86 Western Drive_

Stephenson, OH 60089

Phone No.: _(614)931-3317_

_(   )_

Birth Date: _10/1/56_

Social Security No.: _403-53-3491_

Sex: ☑ Male
☐ Female

Marital Status: ☑ Married ☐ Single
☐ Separated ☐ Divorced
☐ Widowed

Student Status: ☐ Full Time ☑ Non-Student
☐ Part Time

EMPLOYMENT

Employer: _Eastern Linen_

Address: _572 Mehring Way_

Stephenson, OH 60082

Phone No.: _(614)421-3199_ Ext.: _____

Employed: ☑ Full Time
☐ Part Time
☐ Not Employed
☐ Retired

Date: _____

INSURANCE

Primary

Insurance Carrier: _Champ VA_

Policy No.: _321728_ Group No.: _____

Insured: _____

Relationship
to Insured: ☑ Self ☐ Spouse ☐ Child ☐ Other

Co-Pay Amount: _____

Percent Covered: _NA_

Secondary

Insurance Carrier: _____

Policy No.: _____ Group No.: _____

Insured: _____

Relationship
to Insured: ☐ Self ☐ Spouse ☐ Child ☐ Other

Co-Pay Amount: _____

Percent Covered: _____

OTHER

Reason for Visit: _Regular exam_

Known Allergies: _____

Did another physician refer you to our office? ☐ Yes ☑ No If yes, who? _____

Condition Related to: ☐ Auto Accident ☐ Employment Accident ☐ Other Accident

Date Accident Occurred: _____ State Where Accident Occurred: _____

For office use only:

Chart No.: _____ Assigned Provider: _1_ Billing Code: _A_

Signature on File: ☐ Yes ☑ No

Family Care Center
285 Stephenson Boulevard
Stephenson, OH 60089
(614) 555-0100

Provider: Dr. Katherine Yan   **ID #:** 84021   **S.S. #:** 810-99-1110

Patient: Abate, Joe   **Chart #:** ABAJO000   **Document:**

Address: **Phone:**   **Date:** 9/9/98

CODE	DESCRIPTION	X
New Patient		
99201	OF—New Patient Focused	
99202	OF—New Patient Expanded	
99203	OF—New Patient, Complete Physical	✓
Established Patient		
99213	OF—Established Patient Expanded	
99214	OF—Established Patient Routine Exam	
99215	OF—Established Patient Complex	
99211	OF—Established Patient Minimal	
99212	OF—Established Patient Focused	
Procedures		
85007	Manual WBC	
85651	Erythrocyte Sed Rate—ESR	
86403	Strep Test, Rapid	
86585	Tine Test	
87072	Strep Culture	
87086	Urine Culture	
93000	Electroencephalogram—EEG	
93015	Treadmill Stress Test	
90782	Injection	
Other Procedures		

Payments: Received $200, Cash

Diagnosis/ICD-9: Physical exam

Remarks: **Today's Charges:** $ 200.00

Next Appointment: **Amount Paid:** $ 200.00

Family Care Center
285 Stephenson Boulevard
Stephenson, OH 60089
(614) 555-0100

Provider: Dr. Katherine Yan   **ID #:** 84021   **S.S. #:** 810-99-1110

Patient: *Smith, Sarabeth*   **Chart #:** *SMISA000*   **Document:**

Address: **Phone:**   **Date:** *9/9/98*

CODE	DESCRIPTION	X
New Patient		
99201	OF—New Patient Focused	
99202	OF—New Patient Expanded	
99203	OF—New Patient, Complete Physical	✓
Established Patient		
99213	OF—Established Patient Expanded	
99214	OF—Established Patient Routine Exam	
99215	OF—Established Patient Complex	
99211	OF—Established Patient Minimal	
99212	OF—Established Patient Focused	
Procedures		
85007	Manual WBC	
85651	Erythrocyte Sed Rate—ESR	
86403	Strep Test, Rapid	
86585	Tine Test	
87072	Strep Culture	
87086	Urine Culture	
93000	Electroencephalogram—EEG	
93015	Treadmill Stress Test	
90782	Injection	
Other Procedures		

Payments: *Received $200, Check #1299*

Diagnosis/ICD-9: *Physical exam*

Remarks: **Today's Charges:** $ *200.00*

Next Appointment: **Amount Paid:** $ *200.00*

FAMILY CARE CENTER
THINGS TO DO TODAY

Notes:

Checks received on Wednesday, September 9, 1998: 07/08/98 - 09/08/98

From the insurance carrier for Hal Sampson for visit on July 8;

Check #78-9986, $178.50

From the insurance carrier for Samuel Bell for visit on June 29;

Check #561109117A, $90.00

Family Care Center
285 Stephenson Boulevard
Stephenson, OH 60089
(614) 555-0100

Provider: Dr. Katherine Yan   **ID #**: 84021   **S.S. #**: 810-99-1110

Patient: *Ramos, Maritza*   **Chart #**: *RAMMA000*   **Document**:

Address: **Phone**:   **Date**: *9/10/98*

CODE	DESCRIPTION	X
New Patient		
99201	OF—New Patient Focused	
99202	OF—New Patient Expanded	
99203	OF—New Patient, Complete Physical	
Established Patient		
99213	OF—Established Patient Expanded	
99214	OF—Established Patient Routine Exam	
99215	OF—Established Patient Complex	
99211	OF—Established Patient Minimal	✓
99212	OF—Established Patient Focused	
Procedures		
85007	Manual WBC	✓
85651	Erythrocyte Sed Rate—ESR	
86403	Strep Test, Rapid	
86585	Tine Test	
87072	Strep Culture	
87086	Urine Culture	
93000	Electroencephalogram—EEG	
93015	Treadmill Stress Test	
90782	Injection	
Other Procedures		

Payments:

Diagnosis/ICD-9: *Influenza*

Remarks: **Today's Charges**: $ *60.00*

Next Appointment: **Amount Paid**: $

Family Care Center
285 Stephenson Boulevard
Stephenson, OH 60089
(614) 555-0100

Provider: Dr. Katherine Yan   **ID #**: 84021   **S.S. #**: 810-99-1110

Patient: *Bell, Sarina*   **Chart #**: *BELSA000*   **Document**:

Address: **Phone**:   **Date**: *9/10/98*

CODE	DESCRIPTION	X
New Patient		
99201	OF—New Patient Focused	
99202	OF—New Patient Expanded	
99203	OF—New Patient, Complete Physical	
Established Patient		
99213	OF—Established Patient Expanded	
99214	OF—Established Patient Routine Exam	
99215	OF—Established Patient Complex	
99211	OF—Established Patient Minimal	
99212	OF—Established Patient Focused	✓
Procedures		
85007	Manual WBC	
85651	Erythrocyte Sed Rate—ESR	
86403	Strep Test, Rapid	
86585	Tine Test	
87072	Strep Culture	
87086	Urine Culture	
93000	Electroencephalogram—EEG	
93015	Treadmill Stress Test	
90782	Injection	
Other Procedures		
90703		✓

Payments: *Received $80.00, Cash*

Diagnosis/ICD-9: *Laceration*

Remarks: **Today's Charges**: $ *80.00*

Next Appointment: **Amount Paid**: $ *80.00*

Family Care Center
285 Stephenson Boulevard
Stephenson, OH 60089
(614) 555-0100

Provider: Dr. Katherine Yan   **ID #:** 84021   **S.S. #:** 810-99-1110

Patient: *Wong, Jo*   **Chart #:** *WONJO000*   **Document:**

Address: **Phone:**   **Date:** *9/10/98*

CODE	DESCRIPTION	X
	New Patient	
99201	OF—New Patient Focused	
99202	OF—New Patient Expanded	
99203	OF—New Patient, Complete Physical	
	Established Patient	
99213	OF—Established Patient Expanded	
99214	OF—Established Patient Routine Exam	
99215	OF—Established Patient Complex	
99211	OF—Established Patient Minimal	✓
99212	OF—Established Patient Focused	
	Procedures	
85007	Manual WBC	
85651	Erythrocyte Sed Rate—ESR	
86403	Strep Test, Rapid	
86585	Tine Test	
87072	Strep Culture	
87086	Urine Culture	
93000	Electroencephalogram—EEG	
93015	Treadmill Stress Test	
90782	Injection	
	Other Procedures	

Payments: *Received $50, Check #892*

Diagnosis/ICD-9: *Essential hypertension*

Remarks: **Today's Charges:** *$ 50.00*

Next Appointment: **Amount Paid:** *$ 50.00*

FAMILY CARE CENTER
THINGS TO DO TODAY

Notes:

Checks received on Thursday, September 10, 1998:

From the insurance carrier for Hiro Tanaka for visits in August;

Check #199-0015, $125

From the insurance carrier for Lila Saperson for visit on August 11;

Check #348AP11, $40.00

Family Care Center
Patient Information Form

PERSONAL

Name (last, first): _Uzwahl, Surendra_

Address: _15 Main Street_
Stephenson, OH 60089

Phone No.: _(614) 931-3715_
_(   )_

Birth Date: _7/8/57_
Social Security No.: _393-59-4392_

Sex: ☑ Male
☐ Female

Marital Status:
☐ Married   ☐ Single
☑ Separated   ☐ Divorced
☐ Widowed

Student Status:
☐ Full Time   ☑ Non-Student
☐ Part Time

EMPLOYMENT

Employer: _ALX Engineering_
Address: _392 Industrial Pkwy._
Stephenson, OH 60087
Phone No.: _(614) 344-3118_   Ext.: _____

Employed:
☑ Full Time
☐ Part Time
☐ Not Employed
☐ Retired

Date: _____

INSURANCE

Primary
Insurance Carrier: _Blue Cross/Blue Shield_
Policy No.: _393594392_   Group No.: _36_
Insured: _____

Co-Pay Amount: _____
Percent Covered: _80_

Relationship
to Insured: ☑ Self   ☐ Spouse   ☐ Child   ☐ Other

Secondary
Insurance Carrier: _____
Policy No.: _____   Group No.: _____
Insured: _____

Co-Pay Amount: _____
Percent Covered: _____

Relationship
to Insured: ☐ Self   ☐ Spouse   ☐ Child   ☐ Other

OTHER

Reason for Visit: _Ankle hurt in fall_

Known Allergies: _____

Did another physician refer you to our office?   ☐ Yes   ☑ No   If yes, who? _____

Condition Related to: ☐ Auto Accident   ☐ Employment Accident   ☑ Other Accident

Date Accident Occurred: _____   State Where Accident Occurred: _____

For office use only:

Chart No.: _____   Assigned Provider: _1_   Billing Code: _A_

Signature on File: ☐ Yes   ☑ No

Family Care Center
285 Stephenson Boulevard
Stephenson, OH 60089
(614) 555-0100

Provider: Dr. Katherine Yan **ID #**: 84021 **S.S. #**: 810-99-1110

Patient: *Uzwahl, Surendra* **Chart #**: *UZWSU000* **Document**:

Address: **Phone**: **Date**: *9/11/98*

CODE	DESCRIPTION	X
New Patient		
99201	OF—New Patient Focused	✓
99202	OF—New Patient Expanded	
99203	OF—New Patient, Complete Physical	
Established Patient		
99213	OF—Established Patient Expanded	
99214	OF—Established Patient Routine Exam	
99215	OF—Established Patient Complex	
99211	OF—Established Patient Minimal	
99212	OF—Established Patient Focused	
Procedures		
85007	Manual WBC	
85651	Erythrocyte Sed Rate—ESR	
86403	Strep Test, Rapid	
86585	Tine Test	
87072	Strep Culture	
87086	Urine Culture	
93000	Electroencephalogram—EEG	
93015	Treadmill Stress Test	
90782	Injection	
Other Procedures		
73600	*Ankle X ray, AP & Lat*	✓

Payments:

Diagnosis/ICD-9: *Sprain — No cast*

Remarks: **Today's Charges**: *$ 190.00*

Next Appointment: **Amount Paid**: $

Family Care Center
285 Stephenson Boulevard
Stephenson, OH 60089
(614) 555-0100

Provider: Dr. Katherine Yan   **ID #**: 84021   **S.S. #**: 810-99-1110

Patient: *Bell, Jonathan*   **Chart #**: *BELJO000*   **Document**:

Address: **Phone**:   **Date**: *9/11/98*

CODE	DESCRIPTION	X
	New Patient	
99201	OF—New Patient Focused	
99202	OF—New Patient Expanded	
99203	OF—New Patient, Complete Physical	
	Established Patient	
99213	OF—Established Patient Expanded	
99214	OF—Established Patient Routine Exam	
99215	OF—Established Patient Complex	
99211	OF—Established Patient Minimal	
99212	OF—Established Patient Focused	✓
	Procedures	
85007	Manual WBC	
85651	Erythrocyte Sed Rate—ESR	
86403	Strep Test, Rapid	
86585	Tine Test	
87072	Strep Culture	
87086	Urine Culture	
93000	Electroencephalogram—EEG	
93015	Treadmill Stress Test	
90782	Injection	
	Other Procedures	

Payments: *Received $60, Check #8923*

Diagnosis/ICD-9: *Influenza*

Remarks: **Today's Charges**: $ *60.00*

Next Appointment: **Amount Paid**: $ *60.00*

Family Care Center
Patient Information Form

PERSONAL

Name (last, first): _____

Address: _____

_____

Phone No.: ( ) _____

( ) _____

Birth Date: _____

Social Security No.: _____

Sex:
❑ Male
❑ Female

Marital Status:
❑ Married ❑ Single
❑ Separated ❑ Divorced
❑ Widowed

Student Status:
❑ Full Time ❑ Non-Student
❑ Part Time

EMPLOYMENT

Employer: _____

Address: _____

_____

Phone No.: ( ) _____ Ext.: _____

Employed:
❑ Full Time
❑ Part Time
❑ Not Employed
❑ Retired

Date: _____

INSURANCE

Primary

Insurance Carrier: _____

Policy No.: _____ Group No.: _____

Insured: _____

Relationship
to Insured: ❑ Self ❑ Spouse ❑ Child ❑ Other

Co-Pay Amount: _____
Percent Covered: _____

Secondary

Insurance Carrier: _____

Policy No.: _____ Group No.: _____

Insured: _____

Relationship
to Insured: ❑ Self ❑ Spouse ❑ Child ❑ Other

Co-Pay Amount: _____
Percent Covered: _____

OTHER

Reason for Visit: _____

Known Allergies: _____

Did another physician refer you to our office? ❑ Yes ❑ No **If yes, who?** _____

Condition Related to: ❑ Auto Accident ❑ Employment Accident ❑ Other Accident

Date Accident Occurred: _____ State Where Accident Occurred: _____

For office use only:

Chart No.: _____ Assigned Provider: _____ Billing Code: _____

Signature on File: ❑ Yes ❑ No

Family Care Center
Patient Information Form

PERSONAL

Name (last, first): _____

Address: _____

_____

Phone No.: ( ) _____

( ) _____

Birth Date: _____

Social Security No.: _____

Sex: ❏ Male
❏ Female

Marital Status: ❏ Married   ❏ Single
❏ Separated   ❏ Divorced
❏ Widowed

Student Status: ❏ Full Time   ❏ Non-Student
❏ Part Time

EMPLOYMENT

Employer: _____

Address: _____

_____

Phone No.: ( ) _____   Ext.: _____

Employed: ❏ Full Time
❏ Part Time
❏ Not Employed
❏ Retired

Date: _____

INSURANCE

Primary

Insurance Carrier: _____   Co-Pay Amount: _____

Policy No.: _____   Group No.: _____   Percent Covered: _____

Insured: _____

Relationship
to Insured: ❏ Self   ❏ Spouse   ❏ Child   ❏ Other

Secondary

Insurance Carrier: _____   Co-Pay Amount: _____

Policy No.: _____   Group No.: _____   Percent Covered: _____

Insured: _____

Relationship
to Insured: ❏ Self   ❏ Spouse   ❏ Child   ❏ Other

OTHER

Reason for Visit: _____

Known Allergies: _____

Did another physician refer you to our office?   ❏ Yes   ❏ No   If yes, who? _____

Condition Related to: ❏ Auto Accident   ❏ Employment Accident   ❏ Other Accident

Date Accident Occurred: _____   State Where Accident Occurred: _____

For office use only:

Chart No.: _____   Assigned Provider: _____   Billing Code: _____

Signature on File: ❏ Yes ❏ No

Family Care Center
285 Stephenson Boulevard
Stephenson, OH 60089
(614) 555-0100

Provider: Dr. Katherine Yan   **ID #**: 84021   **S.S. #**: 810-99-1110

Patient: **Chart #**:   **Document**:

Address: **Phone**:   **Date**:

CODE	DESCRIPTION	X
New Patient		
99201	OF—New Patient Focused	
99202	OF—New Patient Expanded	
99203	OF—New Patient, Complete Physical	
Established Patient		
99213	OF—Established Patient Expanded	
99214	OF—Established Patient Routine Exam	
99215	OF—Established Patient Complex	
99211	OF—Established Patient Minimal	
99212	OF—Established Patient Focused	
Procedures		
85007	Manual WBC	
85651	Erythrocyte Sed Rate—ESR	
86403	Strep Test, Rapid	
86585	Tine Test	
87072	Strep Culture	
87086	Urine Culture	
93000	Electroencephalogram—EEG	
93015	Treadmill Stress Test	
90782	Injection	
Other Procedures		

Payments:

Diagnosis/ICD-9:

Remarks: **Today's Charges**: $

Next Appointment: **Amount Paid**: $

Family Care Center
285 Stephenson Boulevard
Stephenson, OH 60089
(614) 555-0100

Provider: Dr. Katherine Yan   **ID #:** 84021   **S.S. #:** 810-99-1110

Patient:	Chart #:	Document:
Address:	Phone:	Date:

CODE	DESCRIPTION	X
New Patient		
99201	OF—New Patient Focused	
99202	OF—New Patient Expanded	
99203	OF—New Patient, Complete Physical	
Established Patient		
99213	OF—Established Patient Expanded	
99214	OF—Established Patient Routine Exam	
99215	OF—Established Patient Complex	
99211	OF—Established Patient Minimal	
99212	OF—Established Patient Focused	
Procedures		
85007	Manual WBC	
85651	Erythrocyte Sed Rate—ESR	
86403	Strep Test, Rapid	
86585	Tine Test	
87072	Strep Culture	
87086	Urine Culture	
93000	Electroencephalogram—EEG	
93015	Treadmill Stress Test	
90782	Injection	
Other Procedures		

Payments:
Diagnosis/ICD-9:

Remarks:	Today's Charges: $
Next Appointment:	Amount Paid: $

FAMILY CARE CENTER
Dr. Katherine Yan

Date: _____

Patient: _____

Physician's Notes:

_____

_____

_____

_____

_____

_____

_____

_____

_____

_____

_____

_____

_____

_____

_____

_____

_____

_____

FAMILY CARE CENTER

Dr. Katherine Yan

Date: _____

Patient: _____

Physician's Notes:

_____

_____

_____

_____

_____

_____

_____

_____

_____

_____

_____

_____

_____

_____

_____

_____

_____

_____

FAMILY CARE CENTER
THINGS TO DO TODAY

Notes:

FAMILY CARE CENTER
THINGS TO DO TODAY

Notes:

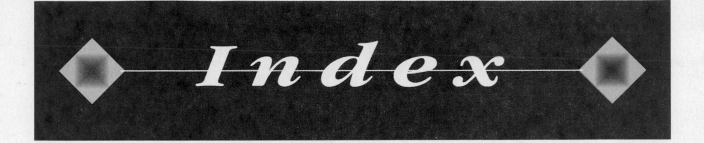

transaction window, illustrated, 100
Personal folder, 70
Phone numbers, entering, 75
POS (Place of Service), 92
Place service codes, common, 95
Policy folders, 71
Practice analysis report, 31, 114, 117, 119:
  defined, 114
  illustrated, 119
Preferred Provider Organization (PPO), 17
Preparing patient statements, 16:
  recording information, 16
Preview report window, 116; illustrated, 116
Primary insurance aging report, 31
Printer button, 116
Printing analysis reports, 117
Procedure, defined, 10, 11
Procedure codes, 16, 28:
  button, illustrated, 32
Program date, defined, 26
Program options, 30
Providers:
  button, illustrated, 32
  defined, 10
  as *MediSoft* list, 28, 31

R

Receivables, defined, 114
Recording information, 16
Records, kept by medical billing assistant, 11-15:
  case, 13
  day sheet, 13
  patient ledger, 13
Reports:
  analysis, 116
  custom, designing, 123
  insurance aging, 117
  lists, 122
  MediSoft, 114-115
  patient aging, 117
  patient day sheet, 115
  patient ledger, 117
  practice analysis, 117
  preview report window, illustrated, 116

printing, 116
printing list, 12
procedure day sheet, 115
types of, 11, 116
viewing, 116
Report options:
  dialog box with lists, illustrated, 122
  illustrated, 32
  in *MediSoft*, 31
  menu illustrated, 32, 122
Restore data option, 30

S

Searching in *MediSoft*, 51-54:
  for chart numbers, 52
  locate button, 53
  for other data, 53
  for patients, 52
  practice, 53
  for procedure code, 54
  resetting, 53
  See also, *MediSoft*
Secondary insurance aging report, 31, 117
Secondary patient ID, defined, 66
Service codes:
  common place, 95
  common type, 95
Show hints button, illustrated, 32
Signature on file, defined, 66
Simulation, patient billing, 147-271:
  procedures manual for, 148-150
  Social Security numbers, entering, 75
  source documents for, 157-271
  step-by-step instructions for, 151-156
Speed key, defined, 26, 35;
  to switch to folder, 77
Status, defined, 130
Status bar, defined, 26
Submenu, defined, 26
Superbill, 11:
  completed, illustrated, 90
  defined, 11
  illustrated, 12
  reviewing a completed, 89
Systems information option, 31

T

Tab key, to move between fields, 95
Tertiary insurance aging report, 31
Tool options, in *MediSoft*, 31
Toolbar, defined, 26; illustrated, 29
Transaction entry window, illustrated, 49, 91, 92:
  case/chart numbers, 91
  entering diagnosis information in, 91
Transactions:
  defined, 88
  entering button, illustrated, 32
  entering option, 30
  kinds of, 88
  processing, 87-107
Type, defined, 66

U

Undo option, 30

V

View backup disks option, 30
Viewing:
  backup files, 58
  data files, 31
  reports, 116

W

Walkout receipt, 93; illustrated, 94
Window, defined, 26
Window option, in *MediSoft*, 31

Z

Zoom buttons, 116; illustrated, 116
Zoom to 100%, 116
Zoom to width of page button, 115